A GUIDE TO LIVING

integrative
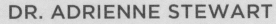
HEALTH

VOLUME 1

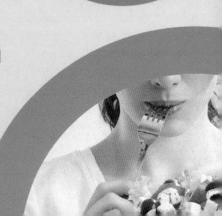

DR. ADRIENNE STEWART

DR. ALAN CHRISTIANSON

DR. LINDA KHOSHABA

DR. SAMAN REZAIE

Printed in the United States of America

First Printing, 2014

ISBN-13: 978-1497309852
ISBN-10: 1497309859

Integrative Health Care Publishing
9200 East Raintree Drive #100
Scottsdale, AZ 85260
www.myintegrativehealth.com
(480) 657-0003

Graphic Designer: Katie Mattson
Editors: Twila Camp and Jennifer Gaston
Cover Designer: Damonza

Because of the dynamic nature of the Internet, any web addresses or links contained in this book may have changed since publication and may no longer be valid.

Integrative Health: A Guide to Living Well is not intended as medical advice. Its intention is solely informational and educational. Please consult a medical or health professional should the need for one be indicated. The information in this book lends itself to self-help. For obvious reasons, the authors and publisher cannot take the medical or legal responsibility of having the contents herein considered as a prescription for everyone. Either you or the physician who examines and treats you must take the responsibility for the uses made of this book.

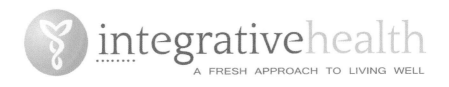

integrativehealth

A FRESH APPROACH TO LIVING WELL

We dedicate this book to YOU and honor your journey to living well.

CONTENTS

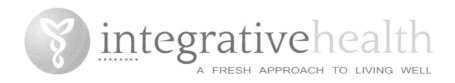

A FRESH APPROACH TO LIVING WELL

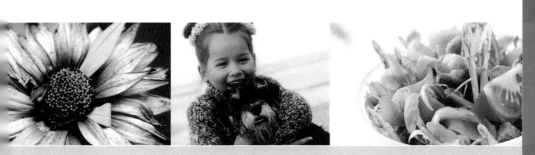

Introduction

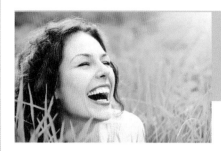

PREFACE

Why we created this book:
Life gets busy – so busy that even when we want to read a great article about health and wellness, we don't always have the time. We promise ourselves that we will come back to it when we can, but months later we can't quite remember where to find it.

We understand. Life gets busy for us, too. That's why we created this book, a compilation of our most recent articles in one place. We want to make it convenient, even fun, to pick it up and read them or share them with family and friends. Our mission is to empower you with the information and tools you need to stay healthy and the wisdom to seek advice when issues arise.

In this book you will find:
- A compilation of our best articles, all in one place
- Some of the most common questions from our patients
- Powerful information to transform your health

We cover topics that are important to you:
- Balancing your life
- Managing your mood
- Increasing your overall health
- Optimizing your hormones
- Exploring seasonal topics
- Increasing your quality of nutrition
- Understanding which foods to eat and which ones to avoid
- Improving your inner and outer beauty
- Managing detox
- Thriving through pregnancy

Health in life is what keeps us going. It is the foundation of everything we do – helping us fulfill our purpose in life, be the best parents to our children, or spend those last remaining years energized and vibrant.

Health is what allows us to do the things that bring us joy and happiness. We are honored to support you and to provide A Guide to Living Well.

ACKNOWLEDGEMENTS

I am forever grateful to my family and friends who have influenced and supported me along my journey to become, and grow as, a naturopathic doctor. I am very blessed to have my amazing newborn Jazlyn, husband Derek, parents Marla and Robert, sister Crystal, and extended family Chris, Grace, Lukas, Rose, Darrell, Brandon, Jennifer, Dean, and Estella. I also want to thank all my patients, mentors, colleagues, Dr. Christianson, and our amazing team at Integrative Health. I truly love what I do, and am honored that I can help others live healthy and happy lives.

Dr. Adrienne Stewart

For the completion of this book, I would like to acknowledge the following people: Dr. Adrienne Stewart, for her vision in initiating this project and her unwavering focus in seeing it to completion; my parents, Glen and Vivian Christianson, for giving me a love of learning and confidence in my ideas; and my beautiful family, Kirin, Celestina, and Ryan, for giving me joy and meaning. I would also like to acknowledge the amazing team at Integrative Health: Miranda, Drs. Khoshaba, Rezaie, Russell, Swanick and Stewart; Ashley, Celia, Easton, Jamie, Jennifer, Kim, Mary, Melissa, Michele, Sharon, and Tipton, for sharing the rewards and the process.

Dr. Alan Christianson

It is a true blessing that I can help my patients, friends and family live healthier and happier lives with the knowledge that naturopathic medicine provides. I would like to thank all of these individuals for allowing me to play a part in their journey to optimal health. I would like to thank my amazing husband, Alen, parents Helen and Hawel, and my amazing grandmother, Maria, for always being there for me. In addition, I would like to thank my colleagues at Integrative Health for helping to create and deliver exceptional patient experiences!

Dr. Linda Khoshaba

I want to thank Integrative Health for the opportunity to be a part of this wonderful team and work in this amazing clinic. The staff and fellow docs are wonderful to work with, day in and day out. I would also like to thank my fiancée, Dr. Lauren Beardsley, for all her support in my career, at home, and in life; and finally, my friends and family, who constantly remind me what is truly important in this world.

Dr. Saman Rezaie

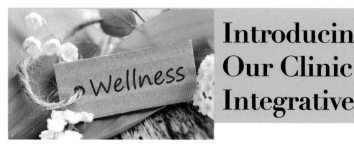

Introducing Our Clinic – Integrative Health

Our Vision:

As the optimal healing community, we co-create integrative solutions that advance your heath and vitality. *We offer a fresh approach.*

Our talented team of vibrant individuals unites as a dynamic and supportive family. *We are passionate about your health.*

Our members act as partners and reward us by honoring their commitments and investing in ideal health.
Your enthusiasm inspires us and motivates others to join our growing team.

We are here to help you feel, look and live better than you ever have before. By diagnosing and treating the root source of your discomfort, your health is no longer a mystery and your healing is simply a matter of fact. Our role is to help you maximize your opportunity to heal, making the most of your treatment process.

The more obstacles to health you choose to remove and benefits to health you choose to adopt, the better your opportunity for success. With a proper diagnosis and treatment protocol, good nutrition, adequate exercise, quality sleep and a healthy frame of mind, your body will begin to heal itself from within. Through this partnership, you can achieve a level of wellness you've never experienced. *This is for life. This is for you!*

Dr. Alan Christianson
Dr. Adrienne Stewart
Dr. Linda Khoshaba
Dr. Soman Rezaie

Dr. Adrienne Stewart

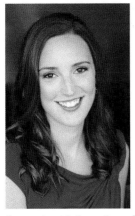

Dr. Adrienne Stewart received her doctorate in Naturopathic Medicine with Highest Academic Achievement from Southwest College of Naturopathic Medicine. She was the first Naturopathic Doctor to attend Dr. Andrew Weil's elective rotation at the Arizona Center for Integrative Medicine. Dr. Stewart's residency at Southwest Naturopathic Medical Center focused on primary care for patients with acute and chronic disease. Prior to medical school, she graduated Summa Cum Laude from the University of Arizona, where she received a Bachelor of Science in Nutritional Sciences with a minor in Chemistry.

When she was a young girl, Dr. Stewart watched her mother struggle with chronic fatigue and fibromyalgia. Going from doctor to doctor, she learned how she did and did not want her family to be treated, and how disease can affect the entire family. These early experiences drew her to become a Naturopathic Medical Doctor.

"Being a naturopathic doctor means getting to do what I love by helping others on a daily basis. I am drawn to helping those with fatigue, thyroid disease, and hormonal shifts. I focus on women's health – as women, mothers, daughters and caretakers, we have innate sense to care for one another."

"I love it when patients come back and tell me how much better they feel. When a patient can finally do what they enjoy in life and spend time with their family, it makes me really happy. I love empowering and teaching patients about their own health and, when they can teach it to someone else, that's when I know I've really made a difference."

Dr. Stewart enjoys dancing and spending time with her family, her husband, Derek, their newborn daughter, Jazlyn, and their dog, Kosmo.

Dr. Alan Christianson

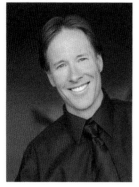

Dr. Alan Christianson is a Phoenix, Arizona-based Naturopathic Medical Doctor (NMD) who specializes in natural endocrinology with a focus on thyroid disorders.

As a child growing up in rural Minnesota, Dr. Christianson had a superior intellect. In fact, he read the encyclopedia from cover to cover before kindergarten. His body, however, told a different story. He struggled with health problems such as epilepsy, poor coordination, and obesity.

Dr. Christianson's nadir occurred in seventh grade when a student directed the class's attention to his rotund physique during gym. Devastated and embarrassed, he became determined to change his health, devoured dozens of nutrition and fitness books over those next few weeks, and discovered at an early age how diet profoundly impacts health.

Over time, Dr. Christianson discovered that medicine didn't have all the answers. Instead, he combined his expertise and insatiable desire for knowledge to teach others how to utilize foods and nutrients for optimal health.

Dr. Christianson gave up sugar and developed a rigorous exercise routine. A year and a half later, the formerly overweight, uncoordinated adolescent was involved in competitive sports and became the class's fastest runner.

He turned that passion into a lifelong endeavor and completed his premedical and nursing studies at the University of North Dakota. He went on to earn his ND with the first graduating class of the Southwest College of Naturopathic Medicine in Tempe, Arizona.

Over time, he discovered that medicine didn't have all the answers. Instead, he combined his expertise and insatiable desire for knowledge to teach others how to utilize foods and nutrients for optimal health.

In 1997, Dr. Christianson broadened that goal by founding Integrative Health, a group of physicians whose philosophy is to "Provide smart, safe, primarily natural and scientific solutions for the entire family to live 'in good health'." The outcome is a more personal, comprehensive approach to health and wellness than simply masking symptoms with pills and procedures.

Along the way, he earned numerous accolades, including 2011 Top Doc recipient in Phoenix magazine. Dr. Christianson co-authored the bestselling book, *The Complete Idiot's Guide to Thyroid Disease*. In addition, he has written *Healing Hashimoto's* and recently completed his next book, which details the relationship between adrenals and obesity. He frequently appears on national TV shows like *The Doctors* and *The Today Show*, as well as in print media, like *Shape Magazine*.

When he's not maintaining a busy practice, his many hobbies include mountain unicycling, marathons, off-road motorcycling, technical rock climbing, and martial arts. He is also a licensed pilot.

Dr. Christianson resides in Scottsdale, Arizona, with his wife, Kirin, their two children, and his six unicycles.

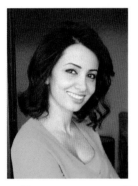

Dr. Linda Khoshaba

Dr. Linda Khoshaba is a licensed Naturopathic Physician (NMD) at Integrative Health in Scottsdale, Arizona. She received her Doctorate from Southwest College of Naturopathic Medicine. Prior to moving to Phoenix, Arizona, Dr. Khoshaba completed her Master's Degree in Health Promotion and Public Health from Brunel University in London, England, where she focused mainly on patient self-management of Type 2 Diabetes Mellitus. She completed her undergraduate degree in Health Sciences (Honors) at the University of Western Ontario, Canada.

Growing up in the Canadian socialized healthcare system, she grew frustrated with the medical solutions and treatments available to her and her family. She has always had a passion to combine health promotion and medicine, and this is the driving factor that led her to become a Naturopathic Physician.

Dr. Khoshaba's specialties include improving digestion, balancing hormones, resolving fatigue, enhancing immunity, diabetes management, and prolotherapy.

Dr. Khoshaba's specialties include improving digestion, balancing hormones, resolving fatigue, enhancing immunity, diabetes management, and prolotherapy. She is a primary care provider who treats all aspects of health and wellness, and she is dedicated to meeting the individual needs of each patient. She is devoted to educating and empowering patients to make lifestyle changes so they can experience life to the fullest. In her spare time, Dr. Khoshaba enjoys traveling and spending time with her family, husband Alen, and dog, Lucky. She has a great appreciation for culture and diversity, as she has studied in three countries and has traveled to more than 20 countries.

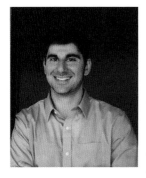

Dr. Saman Rezaie

Dr. Saman Rezaie is a licensed Naturopathic Physician (NMD), receiving his Doctorate from Southwest College of Naturopathic Medicine. Prior to his doctorate, Dr. Rezaie completed a Master's in Molecular Biology from University of Texas at San Antonio (UTSA). During his time at UTSA, he worked with Strength and Conditioning programs for multiple Division I teams at the school and was a Graduate Assistant to the Men's and Women's Tennis teams. He received his undergraduate degree in Biology (pre-dental) from St. Mary's University in San Antonio.

Dr. Rezaie went off to undergrad, and his health dramatically declined in the first semester of college due to diet and inactivity. He gained 25 pounds and was getting sick all the time. He decided to learn more about nutrition, made changes to his diet, and took up distance running. In the second semester of his freshman year, he lost 15 pounds and completely recovered his health. Since then, he has had an avid interest in health through diet and exercise, and its ability to reverse disease and optimize the body. He was able to delve further into the aspects of exercise and understand how diet impacts elite athletes while at UTSA, and at SCNM, he learned numerous therapies to help people reach wellness.

Dr. Rezaie is passionate about sports medicine, pain management, prolotherapy, gastrointestinal concerns, auto-immune disorders, anxiety, depression, and other mental disturbances.

Dr. Rezaie is passionate about sports medicine, pain management, prolotherapy, gastrointestinal concerns, autoimmune disorders, anxiety, depression, and other mental disturbances. He is a general practice physician as well, looking to make the biggest difference in patient health with the smallest possible changes. Dr. Rezaie loves motivating people to achieve health through the power of choice. On his own time, Dr. Rezaie enjoys being with his fiancée, Lauren, league sports, the outdoors with their dog, Logan, and traveling.

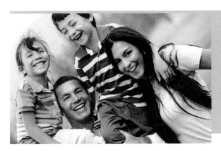

Integrative Health Office Visits

At Integrative Health, our doctors understand that each person's journey may take different avenues to reach a state of optimal wellness. Each patient has his or her unique story, and we are committed to making sure you feel heard, understood, and that you are given the attention you deserve.

What Should I Expect from an Office Visit?
Do you often go to a doctor's appointment feeling rushed and desiring more time with the actual doctor? Our naturopathic physicians dedicate your appointment time to YOU. We take the time to listen to you, share with you our treatment rationale, and answer any questions you may have. Your first visit with your naturopathic doctor will last approximately 60 minutes. Follow-up visits are generally 15 to 45 minutes. This time allows for your doctor to listen to your case and learn about your concerns, health history, family history, and discuss any health obstacles you may need to overcome. Your doctor may then perform a physical exam and order diagnostic tests that are indicated. Retesting and follow-up are often done 1-3 months after initial tests, and then less frequently as symptoms stabilize.

After an assessment of your case, your doctor will work with you to create a treatment plan that is customized specifically for YOU.

Who Goes to a Naturopathic Physician?
Our naturopathic physicians provide healthcare in all stages of life, including healthcare for women, children, families, and seniors. Naturopaths can serve as your primary care physician, or can collaborate or provide adjunctive care with your other healthcare providers. Some patients who visit a naturopathic physician have been to doctor after doctor and are seeking answers and options to their care. They desire a physician who listens and treats not just their physical symptoms, but also their mind and spirit. Other patients who visit a naturopathic physician have little or no symptoms at all. They want to prevent disease and achieve optimal health. Whether you are experiencing an acute illness or chronic disease, our naturopathic physicians can help.

Common Health Benefits:

- Resolve Fatigue and Increase Energy
- Balance Hormones
- Relieve Pain
- Enhance Immunity
- Manage Male Menopause
- Improve Digestion
- Stabilize Thyroid
- Shed Weight
- Relieve Allergies
- Balance Blood Sugar

What is a Naturopathic Medical Doctor (NMD)?
A Naturopathic Medical Doctor (NMD) is a licensed primary care physician who focuses on natural health and wellbeing. The approach to patient care is what distinguishes naturopathic medicine from other medical professionals.

Think of signs and symptoms like a fire alarm in your house. If you hear the fire alarm buzzing, you have two options: 1) you turn off the fire alarm, or 2) you acknowledge the alarm and look for the fire. Option one quickly quiets the buzzing noise, but the fire remains. Option two takes some more investigation, but you can extinguish the fire before it gets too big. Subsequently, the fire alarm turns off and your home is saved from the fire.

Signs and symptoms can be signals to your body that something is out of balance. A naturopathic physician acknowledges your symptoms and listens to what your body may be trying to tell you. Rather than merely suppressing symptoms, a naturopathic doctor searches for the underlying cause.

What makes our process unique?
Our process is unique because of our intuitive listening skills coupled with our seasoned perspective. At Integrative Health, we take the time to learn about you from the inside out. Next, we comprehensively test each of your body's systems to reveal the root source of any issues you may be experiencing. From there, we empower you with the information and resources you need to bring your body back into balance, which heals you from within. It allows you to live your life to its fullest potential, giving your body increased health benefits.

From colds to chronic pain to hormone balancing, our physicians incorporate a therapeutic, diagnostic, counseling, and curative approach. Yes, we provide general practice services, but perhaps most importantly, we strive to provide a fresh approach to living well.

What should I bring with me?
If you take supplements, please bring them or a list of the ingredients. If you have had any relevant tests done, such as blood tests or imaging, arrange to bring copies of the reports with you. If you do not have copies, request that

your doctor's office fax them to us at (480) 657-8693. Please note that some offices may require your written authorization. Feel free to call and confirm that we received your tests a few days before your visit.

Can I take notes or bring a list of questions during my visit?
Of course! The doctors may explain labs, how the body functions, or treatment approaches during your visit at our clinic, so you may find taking notes to be very helpful. Audio recordings may also prove to be valuable. After your visit, the doctor will provide a summary of recommendations as well.

Do you accept insurance?
We are a fee-for-service office and, therefore, do not accept insurance. You are responsible for paying all charges at the time of service. Cash, checks, and major credit cards are accepted. Laboratory testing and treatments are an additional fee – an estimate of those charges will be shared with you prior to performing the tests.

At the end of your visit, you will be provided with an itemized receipt that you may submit to your insurance company to request reimbursement. We can provide you with the information for this process or the names of companies who provide this service. Your individual insurance plan will decide if any of the tests or services performed at Integrative Health are reimbursable.

We are happy to see patients from other parts of the nation and the world.

Currently, we have regular visitors from nearly every continent. Once per year, you can travel to beautiful Scottsdale and have an in-person visit. Between these in-person visits, we can stay in touch via phone, Skype, or Facetime. Over the distance, we can order tests, medications, and send supplements.

Can I be a patient if I don't live in Arizona?
We are happy to see patients from other parts of the nation and the world. Currently, we have regular visitors from nearly every continent. Once per year, you can travel to beautiful Scottsdale and have an in-person visit. Between these in-person visits, we can stay in touch via phone, Skype, or Facetime. Over the distance, we can order tests, medications, and send supplements.

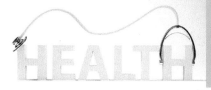

Comprehensive Testing

Your naturopathic doctor is like your personal health detective. We strive to uncover the underlying cause of disease and determine what treatment would be the best fit for you.

A more aggressive discovery rather than a more aggressive treatment

Through comprehensive testing at our clinic, we discover the 'true health' of your body systems, which allows us to address the real source of your discomfort. This discovery empowers you with the comfort of knowing what to do and frees you from the angst of wondering what is wrong.

Yes, our system of comprehensive tests will identify your issues and their causes. What is unique to Integrative Health is the exceptional interpretation and explanation of the findings.

Our physicians' unique perspectives are based on modeling your prognosis within the guidelines of a healthy, vibrant body versus the more traditional approach, which is measured against someone in disease. This innovative solution makes all the difference in your results.

The following is a list of the comprehensive screening exams available at Integrative Health.

SCREENING EXAMS:

Physical Exams
We perform vitals and physical exams based on your particular complaints, such as looking in your ears for an ear infection, looking into your throat for a throat infection (and running a rapid strep test if necessary), listening to your heart for cardiovascular concerns, and conducting complete yearly physicals.

Well Woman Exams with Pap Smear
This is a yearly breast and pelvic exam and may include a Pap smear with HPV testing, if due. This may also include STD or vaginitis testing.

Male Wellness with Digital Rectal Exam (DRE)

This exam is designed to check for problems in the pelvis and lower belly, the gonads and prostate gland in particular, and to check for potential causes of erectile dysfunction.

Physical Medicine Assessment

Aches and pains of the body will be assessed with orthopedic examination and evaluation to help diagnose the underlying cause and help provide a specific treatment plan.

LABS:

As a convenience and service to our patients, we have a lab draw located in our office. There are cash-based prices, and the labs are submitted through your insurance carrier if you have health insurance.

The following are some examples of common labs or panels:

Women's and Men's Wellness Panels

These panels are basic screening labs for possible infections or anemias, liver function, kidney function, and also include results for blood sugar, thyroid function, sex hormones, cortisol, and Vitamin D levels.

Outdoor Allergy Testing

Allergens from the outdoors are inhaled daily into the respiratory tract and can cause allergic reactions locally and systemically. Common allergens found outdoors are trees, molds, grasses, pollens, and pet dander. Once the allergens are identified, a protocol can be put in place to reduce your sensitivity to them and eliminate your symptoms.

NMR (nuclear magnetic resonance) or VAP Lipid Panel

The atherosclerotic culprit is LDL particle number, not LDL cholesterol. This test provides a more accurate picture of cardiovascular (CVD) risk than the standard lipid panel.

MTHFR (methylenetetrahydrofolate reductase) genetic defect

The defective enzyme doesn't break down folate vitamins properly, which may cause high homocysteine, increase your risk of coronary heart disease, blood pressure conditions, depression, thyroid disease, risk of dementia and also inhibit your breakdown of toxins and heavy metals.

Others:

- Autoimmune Panel
- Arthritis Panel
- Celiac Panel
- DTect Dx Breast Cancer Testing
- EBV and CMV Panel
- Hormone Panel
- H Pylori Test
- Hepatitis Panel
- N-Telopeptide (NTx) Bone Marker Test
- Thyroid Panel

IN-OFFICE LABS:

Urine Analysis (UA)
A urine analysis test looks at many properties of a urine sample to help diagnose urinary tract infection, kidney disease, diabetes, and many other conditions.

Candida Testing
Candida albicans is a normal organism that lives in our GI tract. The normal balance of intestinal flora can be disrupted by aggressive use of antibiotics, high sugar intake, and certain types of medications, illness, and diabetes. With candidiasis, symptoms can include fatigue, vaginitis, allergies, foggy brain, and other symptoms. We are able to effectively treat candidiasis based on accurate testing.

Rapid Strep
The rapid strep test is used to determine if a sore throat is "strep throat," caused by group A streptococcus. A swab is rubbed against the back of your throat and tonsils and results are given within minutes.

Others:
• Fecal occult
• Pregnancy
• TB skin testing

SPECIALTY LABS:

Adrenal Stress Testing
Adrenal stress tests provide a comprehensive 24-hour assessment of adrenal function, which is crucial because adrenal stress and/or exhaustion can be at the root of numerous physical and mental health concerns.

Food Sensitivity Testing
The connection between food and symptoms are often overlooked and attributed to another disease or condition. The symptoms from food allergies could be minor, but over time they can develop into more serious issues such as arthritis, chronic fatigue, indigestion, cardiovascular disease, autoimmune disorders, and many others.

Heavy Metal Testing
Patients with chronic illness or exposure to heavy metals can benefit from having their levels assessed with a challenge test. A treatment plan is then created to address toxicity so that the toxic burden of the body is reduced, allowing the body to function optimally.

Stool Analysis Testing
Proper gastrointestinal function is needed to absorb nutrients, eliminate toxins, and for overall health. The gastrointestinal tract has a relationship with the immune and neurological systems. The flora in the GI tract has a big

impact on all of this. Making sure that appropriate levels of beneficial bacteria versus yeast, parasites, and dysbiotic bacteria are in place has a huge impact on your health.

- Beneficial, dysbiotic, and pathogenic bacteria
- Parasites
- Yeast

Mental Health Neurotransmitter Testing

Excessive or deficient neurotransmitters can be the cause for many mood, memory, and behavioral disorders. Once you find out which neurotransmitters are out of range, amino acid, vitamins, and minerals can be used to neuromodulate them.

- Serotonin
- Dopamine
- GABA

Nutrient Testing

Integrative Health offers several different nutritional panels. They are designed to test for amino acids, minerals, micronutrients and vitamins. By finding your specific nutritional profile, your doctor can tailor a supplement protocol to rebalance excessive and deficient nutrients.

Metabolic Analysis Testing

Your individual resting metabolic rate (RMR) is measured through oxygen uptake (VO2). This is a more accurate tool for weight management because it is based on how many calories you actually burn during a day. Once your RMR is calculated, your body fat is measured through bioelectrical impedance analysis (BIA). Your doctor will then customize a diet plan for you based on your requirements.

Referrals

We have a great list of other health professionals who may be appropriate additions to your health team. This may include referrals for screening colonoscopies, full body skin exams, or dental exams.

Imaging orders may include:

- **Thyroid Ultrasounds** – an imaging method to examine the physical structure of the thyroid when it is over or under-functioning.
- **Bone Density (DEXA)** – low-dose x-rays are used to evaluate the risk of fractures.
- **Mammograms** – an X-ray of breast tissue is taken to evaluate for cancer in women that have no signs or symptoms or after a lump, sign, or other symptom of the disease is found.
- **Breast Ultrasounds** – screening exam where a device using sound waves is used to evaluate dense tissue or suspicious areas from a mammogram.
- **Coronary Artery Plaque Testing** – testing that is minimally invasive to look at the extent of occlusion of the coronary arteries.

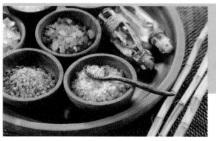

Treatment Options

Each person and each body are unique. Experience our fresh approach to living well.

Naturopaths have the training and scope of practice to order prescription and compounded medications. However, the emphasis of naturopathic treatment is the use of natural healing agents. We often say that we have more tools in our toolbox to choose from. Naturopaths are the only primary care physicians clinically trained in a wide variety of natural medicines and therapies in conjunction with pharmaceutical medications. After evaluating each patient, our naturopathic doctors may use any of the following tools to create your individualized treatment plan:

Acupuncture and Traditional Chinese Medicine:
With origins in China well over 2,500 years ago, acupuncture has received tremendous attention in the past few years from numerous studies demonstrating its effectiveness in providing pain relief. Acupuncture uses sterile, hair-thin needles that are inserted into specific anatomical points in the body.

The goal of acupuncture is to activate the natural, self-healing abilities of the body. It can also strengthen and support the body to prevent future illness and disease. Qi (pronounced *chee*) is energy that flows through meridians as an invisible current, energizing, nourishing, and supporting every cell, tissue, muscle, and organ. A blockage or imbalance in Qi can manifest into various signs and symptoms. Acupuncture helps balance Qi so that healing can occur.

Acupuncture has been used for fibromyalgia, nausea and vomiting due to chemotherapy, smoking cessation, addiction, stroke rehabilitation, headache, menstrual cramps, tennis elbow, myofascial pain, osteoarthritis, low back pain, carpal tunnel syndrome, and asthma, to name a few.

Allergy Relief:
Allergies include reactions to foods and/or outdoor environmental allergens. Food allergies and sensitivities are tested to determine if there are abnormal immune responses to specific foods. Most common food allergies and

sensitivities include dairy, wheat/gluten, eggs, corn and soy. Occasionally, there are sensitivities to even healthy foods, such as fruits and vegetables. Once we have your results, we help you create an individualized diet plan so that you can avoid these foods, repair the gut, and decrease inflammation and irritation to the entire body.

Outdoor Environmental Allergy Testing

Our doctors can also test for outdoor environmental allergies through a simple blood test and treat them with a flavorless spray, without shots or skin tests. Sublingual Immunotherapy (SLIT) helps to treat the cause of the allergy instead of just treating the common symptoms such as runny nose, itchy or watery eyes, and sneezing. Immunotherapy is designed to gradually desensitize the immune system to specific allergens. Patients receive small doses of a specific allergen(s) – not enough to cause a full-blown allergic reaction, but enough to build up a tolerance. Not only does this help allergies, it also calms and strengthens your immune system. Those with autoimmune thyroid disease have better hormone control from the immune repair. Those with frequent colds, flus, asthma, or sinus infections get ill less often.

Biopuncture Therapy:
Biopuncture injections are natural treatments to relieve pain. Biopuncture uses microdoses of natural medicines like arnica, chamomilla, echinacea, cuprum, vitamin B12, Traumeel® or Zeel®, to address the underlying cause of chronic pain and trigger your body's self-healing process.

Biopuncture can address multiple types of pain, including joint pain, muscle pain, neck, shoulder, and back pain, as well as pain from sports injuries, whiplash, tendonitis, sacroiliac pain and tension headache. With biopuncture, chronic inflammation can be reduced, immune function improved, and general detoxification pathways cleared.

Because the biotherapeutic injections are in microdoses, there are no known side effects.

Environmental Medicine and Chelation Therapy

Heavy Metal Detox, or Chelation Therapy, is the administration of chelating agents to remove heavy metals from the body. Chelation for heavy metals is performed intravenously or through oral supplementation with agents designed to target the metal or metals that are at elevated levels.

Environmental Medicine and Chelation Therapy:

Heavy Metal Detox, or Chelation Therapy, is the administration of chelating agents to remove heavy metals from the body. At risk are people who are frequently exposed to large amounts of chemicals, including pesticides (farmers, pest control), paint (auto mechanics, house painters, print shops), and hair dyes (hair stylists). However, a toxic burden can accumulate with simple daily activities such as breathing, eating, and drinking.

Some patients are affected because they grew up near dump sites, or near rivers that were heavily polluted. Most have slower detoxification pathways and have more accumulation from everyday chemical exposure. Symptoms of heavy metal poisoning are neuralgias, increased chemical sensitivities to perfumes or odors, headaches, and other symptoms. Chronic illnesses are also associated with toxicity exposure such as allergies, asthma, diabetes, cognitive difficulties and hormonal imbalances.

After testing to determine the levels and types of heavy metals that may be present, nutrient recommendations and a schedule for chelation therapy will be made. Chelation for heavy metals is performed intravenously or through oral supplementation with agents designed to target the metal or metals that are at elevated levels.

Homeopathy:

Homeopathy is a safe, gentle and effective system of medicine that uses minute doses of a natural substance to induce healing. There are thousands of different homeopathic remedies and, when a patient takes their correct remedy, it increases resilience to stressors and stimulates the body's innate healing capacities. Homeopathic medicines have an effect not only on the body, but also the mind. They are FDA regulated and safe for most everyone, including infants, children, pregnant and nursing women, patients taking multiple pharmaceutical drugs, and the elderly.

Hormone Replacement Therapy:
Our doctors focus on restoring hormones to the normal levels found in your mid-thirties, and focus on both optimal laboratory ranges and your symptoms. Our areas of expertise include:

Testosterone: For both men and women, healthy levels of testosterone maintain peak sexual function, good energy levels, and high exercise capacity. Testosterone can be restored by injections, topical creams, or subdermal pellets.

Estrogen: Given only to women, estrogen stops hot flashes, vaginal dryness, and can reverse memory loss. It can also improve some headaches and sleep disturbances. We give this by injections, topical creams, capsules, or subdermal pellets.

DHEA: When DHEA declines for men or women, the immune system becomes weaker and blood sugar becomes less stable. We give this by pill or topical cream.

Progesterone: Progesterone is for PMS, irregular periods, and painful menses. These symptoms are effectively treated by this hormone, which can be administered either by a topical cream or pill.

Intravenous Micronutrient Therapy or Intramuscular Injection Boosters:
This is the therapeutic use of vitamins, minerals, amino acids, and antioxidants administered directly into the bloodstream. The advantage is that an IV can bypass the gastrointestinal system, where many nutrients may get "lost" due to a poor digestive system. In addition, higher amounts of certain nutrients can be administered in a healthy, safe manner. This is highly effective for acute cold/flu, various levels of pain, athletic recovery, gastrointestinal issues, detoxification, and more.

Lifestyle Coaching:
A therapeutic lifestyle means living your life in a way that will enhance your health, enabling you to achieve optimal function of your body, mind, and spirit. This balance can fight off disease and the signs of aging. Our doctors at Integrative Health can help find the underlying obstacles to your health and recommend great treatment options towards good health.

Lifestyle Coaching

A therapeutic lifestyle means living your life in a way that will enhance your health, enabling you to achieve optimal function of your body, mind, and spirit.

Natural Pharmacy with Supplements and Botanical Medicines:
At the Integrative Health Natural Pharmacy, we have selected and formulated the highest quality natural supplements, botanical tinctures, and specialty products available. We proudly offer the very best in vitamins and supplements for the entire family, each personally selected by our physicians.

We are happy to assist with call-in refills on your supplements and, when needed, mail your products to you.

Natural Primary Care Medicine

From colds to chronic pain to hormone balancing, our physicians incorporate therapeutic, diagnostic, curative care, and counseling to address your healthcare needs.

Natural Primary Care Medicine:
From colds to chronic pain to hormone balancing, our physicians incorporate therapeutic, diagnostic, curative care, and counseling to address your healthcare needs. We provide family practice or general practice (GP) services. Primary care services include routine physical exams, health promotion and disease prevention, diagnosis and treatment of acute and chronic illnesses.

Nutritional Evaluation and Consultation:
Everything we eat provides the nutrients and resources our bodies need to thrive. Some nutrients the body can make itself. Others have to be consumed through food. If we aren't eating them, then they aren't available for our health and wellness. Many of these nutrients aren't just added bonuses; they are essential nutrients we need to function on a daily basis.

Nutrition isn't just about eating healthier, although that's a large part of it. It is also about getting the most nutritional value from the foods you are eating. Things that can compromise the body's ability to absorb nutrients are illnesses of the digestive system such as Celiac Disease, Crohn's, IBS, damage to the digestive system due to repeated use of antibiotics, pharmaceuticals, chronic stress, long-term food sensitivities, and inflammation in the gut. Once these issues are addressed, you can begin healing your gut for optimal health. Not only will this help your body absorb more nutrition, it will help you feel and look your best. When you start to increase the nutrition in your diet, you might find that you have more energy, glowing skin, thick hair and nails, and an increased sense of wellbeing.

Physical Medicine:
This is the treatment of disease and injury by manipulation, massage, trigger point release, active release, stretching, heat, ice, and exercise. This therapy can be very beneficial for acute and chronic injuries, and is usually done in a series of treatments to allow the body to return to health.

Prolotherapy and Platelet Rich Plasma:
Prolotherapy is an innovative injection therapy that uses a solution of dextrose (sugar water) to increase blood supply and your own natural healing components to a specific area. Small amounts are injected into a ligament or tendon where it attaches to the bone, creating a controlled inflammatory reaction and encouraging that area of the body to heal itself.

Physical Medicine

This is the treatment of disease and injury by manipulation, massage, trigger point release, active release, stretching, heat, ice, and exercise. This therapy can be very beneficial for acute and chronic injuries, and is usually done in a series of treatments to allow the body to return to health.

PRP is blood plasma containing concentrated platelets with growth factors, which are vital to the initiation and acceleration of tissue repair. These proteins increase stem cell production to launch connective tissue healing, bone regeneration and repair, promoting development of new blood vessels and stimulating the wound healing process.

It is a technique that reactivates the healing process of the body by injecting a mildly irritating substance - commonly a somewhat concentrated sugar solution, along with the painkiller lidocaine - into the injured area to stimulate a temporary low-grade inflammation. In effect, prolotherapy tricks the body into initiating a healing response. This can be used for both acute and chronic injuries. Prolotherapy is usually a series of treatments that are minimally invasive and cost effective to heal you back to 100%.

Thyroid Disease Diagnosis and Management:
Thyroid disease is a commonly undiagnosed cause of obesity, depression, fatigue, constipation, hair loss and chronic pain. Our doctors are uniquely gifted in the detection of this disease. Many cases are only diagnosed after symptoms have been present for years. Our doctors are also able to treat

it with natural forms of thyroid, helping your gland work better on its own. The founder of Integrative Health, Dr. Alan Christianson, co-authored *The Complete Idiot's Guide to Thyroid Disease* and authored *Healing Hashimoto's: A Savvy Patient's Guide.*

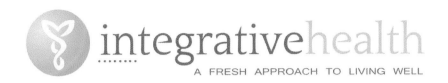

integrativehealth

A FRESH APPROACH TO LIVING WELL

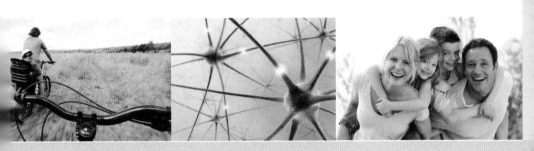

Chapter 1: Life & Mood

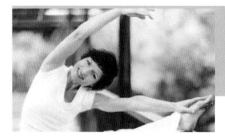

Healing with Passion and Purpose

By Dr. Adrienne Stewart

To fully experience lasting health, we must embrace a lifestyle that supports our minds, bodies, and spirits. Making changes, even positive ones, can be challenging. It takes passion, purpose, and support to make it through the hard times.

After years of helping others achieve optimal health, here are a few suggestions to help you on your own healing journey.

Make health a priority
Empowering our health starts with actively making the time for it, rather than waiting until we find the time. Start by blocking off hours in the day for things like exercise, healthy cooking, journaling, and good quality sleep. It will take discipline not to cut into this time. Whenever you are tempted, remember that you are worthy of having this time to care for yourself.

Define personal health goals
Write down your short and long-term health goals, and be sure to express them using positive language. Share these goals with everyone on your healthcare team, especially your physician. Make a list of things you already do that support your health, and a list of things that would take you one step further. When making your long-term goals, make sure to keep your expectations realistic. Health is a journey to find physical, mental and spiritual balance, so take it in stride and celebrate your milestones along the way.

Review treatment options
Talk to your doctor about all your treatment options. At Integrative Health, we go over different approaches to healing, along with their risks and benefits, to help our patients make informed decisions that are best for them. Together, we may choose one avenue over another, such as botanical medicine, homeopathy, natural hormone replacement, or pharmaceuticals. Our patients find a sense of security in knowing that there are other treatment options to move to in the future.

Determine your commitment level
Regaining health can often mean making lifestyle changes. It is important to decide if you are interested in a short-term program that may address a

portion of good health, or changes that will require long-term commitments for optimal health. It is important to be honest and communicate this to your physician. To address underlying causes of illness, it might require changes to your diet, daily activities, exercise routine, and stress management techniques. Ask yourself what changes you are honestly willing to make, so that you can be truly committed to them.

Identify potential obstacles

The journey towards empowering health will have obstacles. By thinking about them ahead of time, we can line up the support and resources needed to succeed. To start, make a list of habits or behaviors that will have to change for your optimal health. List any barriers such as lack of time, financial resources, or support. Next to each obstacle, brainstorm the tools or resources needed to successfully overcome it.

Gather your support group

We all need support as we build our new, passionate, healthy lives. Make a list of people who will fully support these new goals. Include family members, friends, your physician, and every member of your healthcare team. It's important that each member resonates with your health goals. If someone is not positive about them, try not to rely on that person for encouragement or support. Truly supportive people will help keep you accountable, encourage regular checkups and screenings, be interested in hearing about your progress, and celebrate milestones.

Find a purpose for achieving health

What keeps us motivated and passionate about taking care of ourselves is having a purpose for achieving optimal health. Health is the foundation for everything we do. It can provide us the energy to be the best parents we can be, or the ability to truly enjoy our remaining years. Finding a purpose and a reason to stay healthy will give us the motivation to keep going on our healing journey.

Every journey needs a guide

The doctors at Integrative Health can provide primary care or work with other health professionals as part of a healthcare team. As Naturopathic Doctors, we support our patients by listening to their individual needs and by taking into account the whole person - body, mind and spirit. We encourage every patient to become passionate about their health, and give them the resources and support they need to succeed.

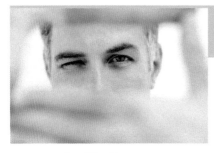

Stress Relief

By Dr. Saman Rezaie

Everybody is looking for stress relief from the constant assault of decisions, events, and relationships that make up everyday life. How can you get some relief? What if the answer was not about relief, but management for the stressors from daily life? Imagine that you are not reacting to stress, but that you have a plan in place to live a more empowered life.

The most important thing to figure out is where your stress is coming from. We can have a lot of answers like work, kids, finances and family, but is this the root of where the stress is coming from? Perhaps the unrealistic mental, emotional and physical demands that we place on ourselves are where we are generating stress. This causes hormones, such as cortisol and neuropeptides, to be released, flooding your body and creating a stressful physical state. First, understand you are creating expectations on yourself that become the stress you are experiencing.

Where is your stress coming from?

First, understand you are creating expectations on yourself that become the stress you are experiencing.

Next, you want to eliminate as much unnecessary stress as possible. It starts with realizing what aspects of life we control and what aspects we do not. Once you let go of the things that are beyond your control, you relieve so much of the added mental and emotional stress you place on yourself. You can then start to focus on the things that you do control. Your thoughts, words, actions, and habits should become the focus of your attention. Start to influence these aspects of your life, and you will become more empowered and feel less worried about everything that is out of your control. The next step is to avoid things that are very stressful to you. Certain places and people can be more than you can handle at times. Remove yourself from these things as much as possible to reduce the amount of unnecessary stress load you experience. By making that decision, you create space for yourself and feel better about your environment.

When looking at the things that create stress for you, try to get some perspective about the situation by reframing it. Take the event and think about how this will impact you, in one month, one year, and even one decade. Is it that important or detrimental to your life? Being able to take any situation and look at it from another view can change how you are feeling about it and, more importantly, how you are reacting to it. With this new perspective, you can focus again on the things that you do control. Now you are ready to more effectively respond to the situation.

To give yourself the best chance at managing stress, it has to start with YOU. This is where you want to make sure you are eating a healthy, balanced diet. This starts with breakfast and continues on with meals throughout the day. Keeping your blood sugars even helps you to handle stress better and have a clear mind. The next thing to add to your routine is regular exercise. If you have an exercise regimen in place, great! If you are lacking in this area, look to start with 30 minutes of mild to moderate activity 3 times per week. Exercise will help alleviate built-up tension, sharpen your mind, and give you a nice endorphin high. Working out should help initiate the next major component of health - sleep. Getting seven plus hours of shuteye a night is needed for recovery and function the next day.

The last thing is to have FUN! This is fun-damental to living a happier life. Doing hobbies you enjoy, having social time with people who brighten your life and stopping to smell the flowers will allow you to be more centered. Putting yourself in this state allows you to fun-ction at a more optimal level and not experience so much stress.

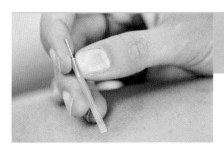

Acupuncture for Depression

By Dr. Adrienne Stewart

Many practitioners of Traditional Chinese Medicine use acupuncture to treat depression because of the gentle and holistic nature of the treatment. Acupuncture is the use of very thin sterile needles placed into various points on the body to help balance the flow of energy, which the Chinese call Qi. This life force energy flows through 12 meridians, or pathways, throughout the body. Each meridian is associated with major organs and functional body systems. Qi is composed of two elements, called yin and yang. Yang is masculine energy, thought to be active and full of light. Yin is feminine energy, thought to be passive and dark. These energies need to be in balance and harmony. When they aren't, we become sick with illnesses, including depression. Therefore, rather than merely focusing on the symptoms of illness, health practitioners who use acupuncture for depression focus more on supporting the whole body system. By stimulating the body's vital force and restoring balance to the flow of energy, patients experience improvement in their depression and in their overall health.

Can Acupuncture Help Depression?

There have been many research studies focused on acupuncture for depression. In a recent study, researchers at the Spaulding Rehabilitation Hospital and Harvard Medical School determined that there was a high level of clinical evidence supporting the use of acupuncture to treat depression. The authors analyzed the findings of various studies that focused on women who were pregnant and suffering from depression. Research showed that not only can acupuncture help depression, it is safe enough for both mother and unborn child. This is in stark contrast to conventional treatments for depression, such as antidepressants, which can't be used during pregnancy because of the effect they could have on the baby. Research studies have also shown acupuncture used in combination with antidepressants, such as fluoxetine (Prozac®), create better clinical results than fluoxetine alone.

A typical acupuncture appointment begins with a detailed medical history and a physical exam, if indicated. The needles are so thin that you might not even feel them, except for a slight tingling, heaviness, or a sensation of heat while the qi is being stimulated. An acupuncture treatment usually lasts about 20 minutes. Acupuncture for depression can be a perfect option for those seeking a safe and balanced state of mind.

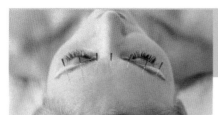

Acupuncture for Anxiety

By Dr. Linda Khoshaba

A commonly asked question is "Does acupuncture work for anxiety?" The simple answer is yes, acupuncture is good for almost every health condition. Acupuncture for anxiety is a common and effective treatment that helps to calm nerves and promote a sense of peace, balance, and restoration. According to Traditional Chinese Medicine (TCM), anxiety is not caused by an imbalance of chemical neurotransmitters, but by the disturbance of Qi. This disturbance is caused by a dysfunction of Qi, and/or a dysfunction in yin and yang within the internal body organs. This is key to the underlying theory of TCM as it explains the pathological, physiological, and aids clinical diagnosis and treatment of disease.

Acupuncture for anxiety focuses on calming the organs by reinforcing and reducing Qi at the meridian point associated with the internal organ. For example, if working on the heart meridian, acupuncture can help anxiety by quieting the spirit and clearing heat. If the problems are within the liver meridian, then treatment would focus on relieving stagnation and draining the liver fire.

How can acupuncture help anxiety?

Acupuncture for anxiety focuses on calming the organs by reinforcing and reducing Qi at the meridian point associated with the internal organ.

You may be wondering if acupuncture help anxiety? Anxiety itself can manifest other symptoms such as sadness, worry, fear, palpitations, insomnia and irritability. Understanding the kind of anxiety can be useful and allows the practitioner to choose specific acupuncture points to make an appropriate and balanced protocol. An average number of points used in acupuncture for anxiety can be anywhere from 10-20 points and is usually performed on both sides of the body. A good treatment duration would be anywhere from 20-30 minutes and would achieve optimal benefits if frequency of treatment was anywhere between 4-6 times per month.

In addition to understanding the symptoms, other useful tools for diagnosis include tongue and pulse diagnosis. An acupuncturist can identify conditions just by looking at your tongue and feeling your pulse. In the case of heart deficiency, a typical tongue would look red at the tip, with red body and teeth marks on the outer edges. The person's pulse may feel weak and wiry. Depending on the organ system causing anxiety, tongue and pulse diagnosis would differ.

Acupuncture for anxiety is a great adjunct to any medical therapy. Not only does it help balance the inner Qi, it also promotes a sense of wellbeing and relaxation.

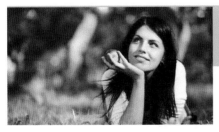

Mind Full or Mindful?

By Dr. Linda Khoshaba

What is Mindfulness?

Mindfulness is the complete state of awareness of the present moment. Easier said than done, right? How many of you would agree that we are either too focused on what we need to get done later in the day, tomorrow or next week or too focused on something that happened a day, week or month, perhaps even years ago? The majority of the time, the human brain is either focused on the past or future, and rarely do we make time or experience total awareness of what is going on in the present moment.

We are often pretty good at identifying physical symptoms in our body, but do we take the time to make sense of the mental symptoms that occur? Mental symptoms can include thoughts, worries, fears, irritability, and so on. Stress and time are usually causes of these mental symptoms. Being mindful means focusing on the present moment and paying full attention to what is going on around you. Here is a simple mindful exercise that you can practice daily. You know what they say about practice... It makes perfect!

Mindfulness Exercise
Before starting the exercise, situate yourself in a peaceful, quiet room and prepare to engage in this exercise for at least 5 minutes. As you start, take a deep breath and focus your attention to the sight, smell, and thoughts of the present moment. Bring your attention and focus to what is going on internally. If you feel that your thoughts are talking to you about either the past or the future, just become aware of this and bring yourself back to the present moment. Keep your focus on your breathing as you inhale slowly and feel your abdomen expand. Gently exhale and feel your abdomen retract back to the original position. Try a series of these breathing exercises for at least 5 minutes and really try to focus on the present moment, enjoying the experience this exercise can bring you. This exercise should ideally be practiced at least once per day, and it is a great way to either start or finish your day. It even makes a great exercise throughout the day to help you relax and feel more in control of your thoughts, emotions and feelings.

Not only can mindfulness help you relax, it can also bring about positive changes in physical symptoms, such as lowering blood pressure, improving sleep, reducing chronic pain, and alleviating an upset stomach. Mental health can also improve with mindfulness, and this is a great therapy for people who suffer with anxiety, depression, obsessive-compulsive behavior, eating disorders, and substance abuse.

Mindfulness allows you to focus on yourself and get a better understanding of your inner senses. It also allow you to get in touch with your emotions and understand them without judgment. The more you can practice this in your daily life, the easier it becomes and the more benefits you will see. It is a technique that has been used for hundreds of years throughout many religions and cultures, because it helps you to shift your thoughts from the future or past back to the present moment. Give it a try and allow yourself the gift of being fully present in this moment!

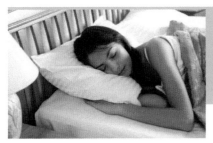

How Sleep Could Make You a Better Person

By Dr. Alan Christianson

A terrible night's sleep can have numerous ramifications the following day. Because you're already running late, you forego breakfast for the drive-thru, where you get a mega-cup of coffee sweetened with sugar or aspartame and a cream cheese-smeared bagel.

Your already frustrating morning commute becomes so much more of a hassle with too little sleep, and you find yourself barking at your assistant for even the slightest misstep. Your eight hours at the office will feel more like 30 getting a root canal.

But poor sleep affects more than your dietary lapses of judgment and bad mood. Getting too little shuteye can also knock your hormones completely out of whack. Let's briefly look at four of those hormones and how they affect you with too little sleep:

Insulin
Poor sleep can make your cells insulin-resistant, stalling fat loss and contributing to cancer, diabetes, and heart disease. Erratic insulin levels also make you more likely to crave (and devour) those chocolate chip cookies your coworker brought in. Couple your blood sugar spike and crash with sleep deprivation, and you have a surefire strategy for lethargy, brain fog, and just generally feeling "off."

Growth hormone
Sometimes called the "fountain of youth" hormone, the growth hormone helps you build muscle and burn fat. Your body makes growth hormones while you sleep, so a lack of sleep can inhibit production of this anti-aging hormone.

Testosterone
Your testosterone levels are highest early in the morning and lowest around 8 p.m. Sleep helps rejuvenate this hormone. In fact, studies show poor-quality sleep leads to low testosterone levels. Therefore, quality sleep is perhaps the best thing you can do to boost testosterone.

Cortisol

Studies show that too little sleep elevates your levels of the stress hormone, cortisol, the next day. You'll hear a lot about cortisol in this article. While cortisol can be beneficial, such as when someone swerves into your lane on the freeway, it is not meant to always be "on." Chronically high cortisol levels mean you're more likely to store fat, break down muscle, and be a cranky mess at the office.

To balance your hormones and mood, I recommend you aim for eight hours of quality, uninterrupted sleep every night. Fortunately, there are a number of simple tactics you can use to make sure you sleep more soundly. Here are 10 of the most effective ones I use with patients:

Take a power nap, not an afternoon siesta

Ah, Sunday afternoon – a time to catch the game on TV or maybe just leisurely do the *Times* crossword. You might also drift into a peaceful slumber. One study showed that a 30-minute nap promotes wakefulness, enhances your performance, and improves cognitive function. It can also boost your testosterone levels. Sleep longer than that, and you risk lying awake at night, staring at the alarm clock and dreading the day ahead.

Clean up your diet

A high-carbohydrate diet can lead to blood sugar spikes and crashes and raise levels of cortisol, which can make you tired during the day and more restless at night. Make every meal high-quality protein, good fats, leafy green vegetables, and high-fiber starches. Snack on nuts, seeds, and nitrate-free jerky. As much as you can, eliminate sugar and other processed carbs from your diet.

Exercise

Studies show exercise can help you get a better night's sleep. Work out in the morning or early afternoon, since exercise too close to bed can leave you wired rather than tired. Reduce the time-consuming cardio for weight resistance and burst training, two very efficient, effective forms of exercise that help you blast fat, boost testosterone, and contribute to solid sleep.

Reduce your stress levels

Stress and lack of sleep are a vicious cycle. Chronic stress elevates – you guessed it! – cortisol, which interferes with sleep. And too little sleep ramps up your cortisol levels during the day. You can't eliminate stress, but you can acknowledge what you can control and let go of the rest. And give yourself a work curfew at night so you don't stumble across your boss's vitriolic email at 10:30 p.m.

Prepare for sleep

Speaking of checking late-night emails, I recommend you turn off all electronics and any other stimulation about an hour before bedtime. Otherwise, you're likely to get caught up in the evening news or online shopping, and before you know it, it's midnight. Have a calming cup of tea, take a hot bath, or try some deep breathing to help you drift into sleep.

Watch the caffeine

A morning cup of organic coffee can get your mind and body going. But if you metabolize it slowly, too much caffeine can interfere with sleep. Keep it to the morning, or better yet, switch to green tea, which provides a caffeine boost without the jittery aftermath. And be very mindful of the nightcap. A shot of whiskey (or whatever your poison might be) might knock you out, but you're likely to wake around 3 a.m. dehydrated and having to urinate. Keep the alcohol to a glass or two with dinner and call it quits.

Zap the snoring

You snore because your airways that connect your nose and mouth to your lungs narrow while you sleep, which increases pressure for sufficient airflow. Studies show being overweight increases your chances of snoring. Sleep apnea, or abnormal or slow breathing while you sleep, also triggers snoring. It can create sleepiness and diminished alertness the following day. Sleep apnea can contribute to hypertension and diabetes. Studies also show that about half the guys who snore suffer erectile dysfunction. If snoring creates a problem for your partner, or you suspect it could be creating health issues for you, talk with your doctor about potential solutions.

Mind Your Stress

Getting sufficient sleep helps restore your adrenals and balance cortisol (your stress hormone) levels.

Check your adrenals

Remember cortisol, your stress hormone I mentioned earlier? When your adrenals over-secrete this hormone, they eventually become burned out. Because your stressed-out adrenals are on hyper-drive, they're secreting cortisol and other stimulating hormones even at night. Being wired before bed can also cause sleeplessness. Getting sufficient sleep helps restore your adrenals and balance cortisol levels. Also consider non-glandular support with key adaptogenic herbs to improve your body's resistance to stress and optimize adrenal function.

Ditto for your testosterone

I mentioned earlier that poor sleep contributes to low testosterone, but studies also show the reverse. Low testosterone can impact your sleep quality and duration. A vicious cycle ensues; too little sleep raises your stress hormone cortisol, further crashing testosterone levels. If you suspect low testosterone contributes to your restless nights, talk to your doctor about testosterone replacement therapy (TRT) and other options.

A sleep aid might be your ticket

If you frequently experience jetlag, erratic bedtimes, and other issues that can impact sleep, consider supplementing with melatonin. Your pineal gland's melatonin secretion declines as you age, and a supplement can help regulate circadian rhythm for a good night's sleep. Herbal remedies to help you sleep better include valerian and chamomile, either as supplements or as a tea.

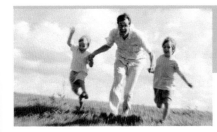

Lifestyle Factors to Health

Here are some general lifestyle factors that can help improve your health:

Environmental Management

Avoid routine applications of insecticides or pesticides to your home or work environment.

Replace air intake filters every month.

Use shower filters to remove chlorine.

Do not exercise near traffic or outdoors on high pollution days.

Use indoor air filtration and ionization systems, especially if prone to allergies or respiratory infections.

Avoid electromagnetic fields coming from cell phones, microwave ovens, computers, electric razors, radio/alarm clocks, hair dryers, electric blankets, television and fluorescent lighting.

Avoid sources of aluminum such as aluminum cookware and anti-perspirants.

Use iron or stainless steel cookware and avoid non-stick items.

Avoid plastic or Styrofoam food containers and do not heat foods in either.

Test your home for lead, especially if you have young children.

Exercise

For general health, include aerobic exercises, like jogging, running, brisk walking, swimming, hiking, cycling, rollerblading or dance, 2 to 6 times a week and strength exercises, like free weights, weight machines, calisthenics, yoga, Pilates, or Qigong 2 to 3 times a week. If weight loss is the goal, walk, jog or run at least 4 miles a day or view exercise charts and calculate what it would take for you to burn 2800 calories weekly. Less is probably not effective.

Mental and Emotional Wellness

Meditate Daily!

Work to maintain good relationships with co-workers, family, friends and loved ones. If this is not successful, consider studying material like Kirchner and Brinkman's *How to Deal with Difficult People* or Eckert Tolle's various books on self and world healing. Also try engaging in psychotherapy such as Cognitive Behavioral Therapy.

Spend time immersed in nature on a regular basis.

If possible, help those in greater need. There is no better remedy for suffering than lessening someone else's.

Engage in regular activities that allow you to experience emotional release. This can come from journaling, music, art, exercise or deep dialogue.

Stay active with any religious or spiritual system of belief you have affinity with.

Regularly allocate time and resources for your favorite recreations.

Learn to see adversity as challenge and see change as opportunity. Pessimists feel smugly assured of their correctness, while optimists are happier. Which choice is better?

Sleep

During sleep our bodies are restored and rebuilt. If left in a dark, quiet room for 10 minutes, would you fall asleep? If so, you are probably sleep deprived. The most restful sleep you can get occurs before midnight. Each minute of sleep before midnight is equivalent to 10 minutes of sleep after midnight. Interestingly, the slant of the sun's rays in the early morning stimulates the production of lithium in our bodies, which is our natural antidepressant. So the old adage, "Early to bed, early to rise makes a body healthy, wealthy and wise" is a very true statement! To help you sleep, keep the room dark, use the bedroom only for sleep and romance, and avoid protein foods after 6 pm.

Sunlight

Spend some time in the sun every day. This is essential for vitamin D, melatonin and serotonin formation. Be careful not to overdo it if you are fair skinned, in a hot climate or not used to being outdoors. Plan for 15 to 30 minutes daily and avoid exposure from 11 am to 2 pm.

Keep Your Intestinal Track Healthy and Clean

Include high fiber foods in your daily diet. Drink water! Take a daily probiotic, and even more often when you are getting sick or if you have taken antibiotics for any reason. Talk to your doctor about colonics.

Supplement Your Diet with Good Nutrients

Because of biogenetic engineering, pesticide use, and the over farming/ grazing of our lands, our food supply today has a lower vitamin and mineral content than ever before. Combine this with a busy lifestyle, which can make it difficult to eat correctly each and every day, and we often miss getting all the nutrients our body needs. Unless you are instructed otherwise by your doctor, it is good to take quality multivitamin and minerals, Omega-3, calcium/magnesium/zinc combo, D3, and a probiotic. If you sweat or exercise a lot, add an electrolyte blend.

A therapeutic lifestyle means living your life in a way that will enhance your health, enabling you to achieve optimal function of your body and mind, as well as fight off disease and the signs of aging. Every day it is up to YOU to make the correct choices towards good health! Choose good foods for your body. Choose healthy thoughts for your mind. Choose to exercise. Choose to have a positive outlook. As you review the above guidelines, highlight areas you need to incorporate into your lifestyle. Read those areas on a daily basis. Choose just one area a month and consciously work to apply it to your life until it becomes a daily routine. We wish you success in your endeavor to achieve optimal health!

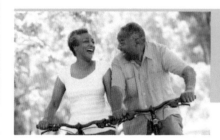

The Healing Power of Relationships

By Dr. Adrienne Stewart

Our health is influenced by the relationships we have in many areas of our life, such as our relationships with food, exercise, friends and family, and even ourselves. Making positive choices in these areas can empower and support our optimal health.

Relationship with Food

Many things can challenge our relationship with food. One of the biggest is the desire to eat for emotional support. We might grab chocolate during times of stress, or overeat when we feel depressed. Another challenge is avoiding fast, inexpensive food that has little nutritional value. When we are pressed for time, we might grab takeout, have pizza delivered, or make boxed foods. Another common challenge is avoiding food sensitivities such as dairy or gluten. It can be difficult to give up foods that have become part of your lifestyle or that you may crave. When our relationship with food is unhealthy, it can sabotage other health goals, decrease our energy, lower our immune system, and work against the body's natural vitality.

One strategy is to be aware of what foods you are eating, when you are eating them, and how you feel before and after the meal. A food diary for one week is an easy way to have a broad overview of what you are eating on a routine basis. The more specific you are with your food diary, the more helpful it will be to assess healthy and unhealthy patterns in your diet.

Relationship with Exercise

Our relationship with exercise is important to our overall vitality. It can be hard to start an exercise routine if it is not already part of your lifestyle. Some people might feel they need to be fit already in order to have a workout routine. However, this misconception is only holding them back. Regular exercise is linked to better health, improved sleep, reduced stress, increased sex drive, and other positive effects. A healthy relationship with exercise starts with attainable goals, such as exercising a few times per week. Keep your motivation high by finding forms of exercise you enjoy, joining a class, or exercising with a friend. Your motivation will improve if you like what you are doing. After you have made exercise a part of your routine, begin challenging yourself to go further each time. This will help you build up endurance, strength and stamina.

Relationship with Friends and Family

It is important to have strong social bonds with family and friends. Not only do your relationships with others provide emotional support, but they also increase your happiness levels and sense of meaning. Social support is especially important for coping with daily stress and significant life changes. Listen to the positive messages friends and family have for you - especially if they are encouraging you to see a doctor to support your health goals. Remember to have fun and enjoy each other as well. Laughter is great medicine.

Life's Relationships

Our health is influenced by the relationships we have in many areas of our life, such as our relationships with food, exercise, friends and family, and even ourselves.

When spending more time with friends and family, be aware of how they make you feel and if they support your overall health goals. Identifying toxic friends or family members will help you know who to count on for support and from whom you may need to distance yourself.

It can be especially difficult if spouses do not agree or support each other with significant changes in their lifestyle. One spouse may decide to stop smoking or eating sugar, while the other does not. Respecting each other's decisions can go a long way to avoiding painful conflict. It is important to talk about your goals, decide how you can support each other, and how best to keep each other accountable.

Relationship with Yourself
The foundation of all relationships begins with the relationship you have with yourself. When your relationship with yourself is off balance, it can make it more difficult to have a healthy relationship with food, exercise, family and friends. Signs that you may be struggling in this area are low self-worth, poor body image, and low self-esteem. These might be signs that you are holding onto regret, anger and fear. If you feel out of balance, it might help to do more things that you enjoy, like journaling, taking a walk, or spending time with friends. It is important to keep in mind that health is a personal journey. Taking time to be present and nurture yourself can help give you the motivation to make healthy choices in all areas of your life.

Ultimately, your health is in your own hands. Being mindful of your relationships in all areas can help empower you to make healthier choices. Remember to create space in your home and life that honors your healing journey, and seek out the support you need to attain better health.

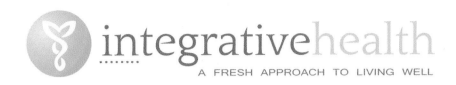

integrativehealth

A FRESH APPROACH TO LIVING WELL

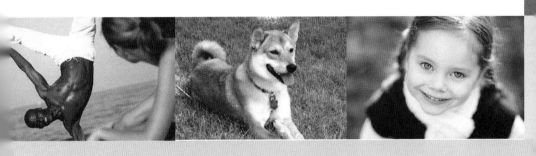

Chapter 2: Health

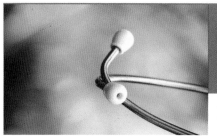

Are You on Track with Your Health Exams?

By Dr. Adrienne Stewart

They say an ounce of prevention is worth a pound of cure. At Integrative Health, we believe prevention is the best medicine. That is why we recommend annual health exams as an essential part of your long-term health goals.

Health exams can often make people feel anxious. The fear of getting unexpected news can keep you from taking action. That is why we work with each patient individually to create a plan that supports them. Our doctors counsel patients on their options, risk factors, and recommended screenings, while supporting them with resources and explanation of lab results.

Here are some key screening areas and why each one is important.

Blood Work and Physical Exams
Routine blood work and a physical exam should be done annually for both men and women. These tests can help your doctor look for things like hypertension, anemia, infections, cholesterol levels, liver and kidney function, blood sugar levels, and thyroid function. Depending on your individual health and treatment plan, your doctor might also test your vitamin D and hormone levels.

Women's Health Screenings
There are some annual tests that are specific to women's health. A Well Woman Exam is recommended yearly and includes a breast exam and pelvic exam to check your uterus and ovaries for problems such as cysts, physical abnormalities, and growths. Both of our female doctors at Integrative Health offer Well Woman Exams.

At the same time as the pelvic exam, we can perform a Pap and HPV test. Many national medical organizations recommend starting Pap exams at age 21 and repeating these tests at least every three years. The Pap test looks for cellular changes on the cervix that might become cervical cancer if not treated. The HPV test looks for the human papillomavirus that can cause these kinds of cellular changes. The HPV test can be done at the same time as the Pap test for convenience and is recommended for all women over 30 years old.

Because breast cancer is the second most common cancer among American women, mammograms are recommended every 1-2 years for women over the age of 40. Clinical breast exams and self-breast exams are recommended routinely. This is when you check for lumps, changes in size or shape of the breast, or any other changes in the breasts or axilla (armpits). We recommend adding a breast ultrasound to your mammogram, especially if you have dense breasts. Dense breasts make it harder for a mammogram to find cancer. Women with breast implants should continue to have mammograms.

There are a few concerns with mammograms that include false-negative results, false-positive results, over diagnosis, overtreatment, and radiation exposure. If you would prefer not to have mammograms, there are other types of screening, including a blood test called dtectDx Breast, and breast thermography. Feel free to talk to our doctors for more information.

Men's Health Screenings

Men's Health

Prostate cancer is the second most common cancer in men in the United States. There are two tests your doctor may order, which are commonly used to screen for prostate cancer.

Prostate cancer is the second most common cancer in men in the United States. There are two tests your doctor may order, which are commonly used to screen for prostate cancer.

The prostate-specific antigen (PSA) test is a blood test for men that can be added to your routine screening blood work. This test is commonly recommended starting at age 50 for average risk. If you are African American or have a family history of prostate cancer, it may be best to start at age 40. A high PSA level does not always mean that a man has prostate cancer. It may be elevated due to other types of prostate problems or because of factors with the test itself. It is important not to test PSA directly after a digital rectal exam or within two days of ejaculation, horseback riding, or biking. In addition, high or low blood sugar and certain medications can interfere with the test. Commonly, if the PSA is initially or slightly elevated with no other symptoms or signs of concern, it is retested in 2-3 months.

The other type of test is a Digital Rectal Exam (DRE) where the doctor inserts a gloved, lubricated finger into the rectum to feel the prostate for asymmetry, lumps, enlargement, or anything else unusual. Either of our male physicians at Integrative Health can perform this screening physical exam.

Bone Health
Healthy bones are essential for aging gracefully and for quality of life. The National Osteoporosis Foundation recommends testing postmenopausal

women, all women over the age of 65, all men over the age of 70, and men between 50-69 years old with a high risk factor profile. The first 5 years post-menopause is the time of most bone loss. At Integrative Health, we recommend getting tested early to have a baseline for comparison and to help determine which bone nutrients or hormonal support may be needed. In addition, if you have higher risk factors (history of smoking, previous fractures, use of corticosteroids, amenorrhea or anorexia), it may be a good idea to screen early as well. To screen for bone mineral density, your doctor can order a Dual-energy X-ray absorptiometry (DXA). This test is used to help diagnose osteopenia or osteoporosis. The frequency for this test is commonly every other year if there are any abnormal results, or every 5 years if there are normal results. Another test is a Nterminal telopeptide (NTX) urine test. This test helps measure the rate of bone turnover and if we need to make any treatment plan adjustments.

Colon Health

If you are 50 or older, getting a colorectal cancer screening test could save your life. Screenings will help detect both polyps, which can turn into cancer, as well as colorectal cancer at an early stage.

The frequency of routine colonoscopies is every 10 years, unless advised more frequently by your gastroenterologist. If you have a parent that was diagnosed with colon cancer, it is recommended that you start getting screened 10 years prior to their age at diagnosis. So, for example, if your father was diagnosed at age 50, it is recommended that you begin your colonoscopies at age 40.

There are other types of screening tests including a High-Sensitivity FOBT (stool test), flexible sigmoidoscopy, double contrast barium enema, virtual colonoscopy, and stool DNA test.

Other Screening Tests

Skin Cancer Screening: Skin cancer is the most common form of cancer in the United States. About 171 people in Arizona die of melanoma every year. Since 1975, the melanoma death rate in Arizona has risen by an average of about 1% per year among residents over the age of 50. At Integrative Health, we recommend getting a yearly screening skin exam from a dermatologist.

Thyroid Screening: If you have thyroid disease, we recommend a yearly screening thyroid ultrasound. Thyroid cancer is one of the few cancers that has increased in incidence over recent years and occurs in all age groups, from young children through seniors. An ultrasound can check for thyroid size, masses or nodules and follow-up screening can monitor for number, size, and stability of nodules if you have them. Thyroid cancer is usually highly treatable when found early.

Sexually Transmitted Diseases: Depending on your risk factors, we also recommend screening tests for sexually transmitted diseases. These risk factors include having unprotected sex, sexual contact with multiple partners, a history of STDs, or abusing alcohol or recreational drugs. If you have symptoms of an STD, it's important to be tested. However, many infections often do not cause any symptoms. Getting tested can put your mind at ease or get you (and your partner) treatment if needed.

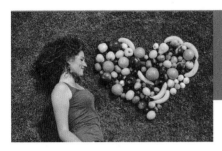

Heart Healthy Habits

By Dr. Linda Khoshaba

Your heart is one of your body's strongest muscles and is responsible for pumping over a billion gallons of blood throughout your circulatory system during your lifetime. What are you doing to make sure this organ is fit to do the job and do it well in your lifetime?

Here are **5 great and simple tips** that you can include in your lifestyle to help you achieve the maximum benefits of having a fit and healthy heart.

1. Eat a diet that is rich in vegetables, fruits, whole grains and fiber
Healthy diets rich in vegetables and fruits provide essential vitamins and minerals such as Vitamin A, Vitamin C, folic acid, potassium, and magnesium. These nutrients help prevent coronary heart disease, maintain good blood pressure, and promote healthy body weight. Eating a variety of vegetables and fruits not only protects your heart, it helps prevent chronic disease.

Heart Health Tip: When making breakfast or lunch, consider substituting lettuce, tomatoes and onions instead of cheese. This is a very simple way to get the extra fiber with fewer calories! Remember, this is all a part of making a difference in your lifestyle.

2. Eliminate unhealthy fats and cholesterol
Unhealthy fats are known as trans fat, saturated fat, and hydrogenated oils. Replace these with monounsaturated fats, such as olive oil, and polyunsaturated fats, such as nuts and seeds. These healthier types of fats will help you maintain a healthy cholesterol level and prevent the risk of atherosclerosis.

Heart Health Tip: Not only do nuts and seeds have great sources of fat, they are also rich in vitamins and minerals and are a great source of protein. Sprinkle a few walnuts, almonds, and sesame seeds on your oatmeal or salad. You can also grind them up and add them into a smoothie.

3. Manage Stress

Stress is when the body tends to go into system overload and compensates by producing physiological changes that can affect the entire body. In addition, prolonged periods of unmanaged stress can cause changes in our thoughts, feelings and behaviors. For example, if you are stressed, this can increase your blood pressure and the incidence of blood clots, thereby increasing your risk for a heart attack. Recognizing the signs of stress is essential in helping you manage it properly.

Heart Health Tip

Not only do nuts and seeds have great sources of fat, they are also rich in vitamins and minerals and are a great source of protein. Sprinkle a few walnuts, almonds, and sesame seeds on your oatmeal or salad. You can also grind them up and add them into a smoothie.

Heart Health Tip: Simply taking control of your breath is one of the most powerful tools at your fingertips. Place one of your palms on your belly. With your mouth closed, take in a deep breath from your nose and feel your belly expand. Exhale slowly and repeat this series for 10 breaths. This exercise, which can reduce your heart rate and blood pressure and promote relaxation, is a great tool that you can incorporate into your daily life.

4. Create a Fun Daily Exercise Plan

Are you getting enough daily exercise? The American Heart Association recommends 30 minutes of daily exercise. You will notice a plethora of benefits from exercise, including improving circulation, reducing inflammation of blood vessels, and keeping cholesterol levels in check. Every little bit of physical activity goes a long way for your heart.

Heart Health Tip: If it is a warm and sunny day outside, consider going for a walk. If at work, incorporate exercise by taking the stairs instead of an elevator. You can also get creative with office equipment, such as using a chair for dips to strengthen triceps, or using an exercise ball as a chair to improve core muscles.

5. Smile

It takes more effort and muscle energy to frown than it does to smile (43 muscles vs. 17). This simple act can improve cardiovascular function and happiness by reducing physiological responses to stress, boosting your immune system and triggering the brain to release serotonin. The power of a smile is contagious, and this will not only benefit *your* health, but can influence someone else's.

Heart Health Tip: Next time you are in a grocery line or in an elevator, go ahead and smile. Test the power of this gesture and pass on the positive heart side effects!

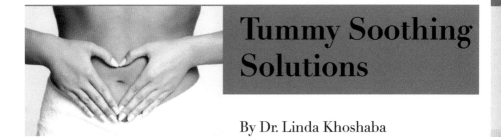

Tummy Soothing Solutions

By Dr. Linda Khoshaba

At some point in your lifetime, you may have experienced some of the following symptoms: reflux, heartburn, gas, bloating, stomach distention, cramps, abdominal pain, diarrhea, constipation, and vomiting.

You may have tried conventional treatments that worked in the short term. These conventional treatments may have ranged from proton pump inhibitors, like Prilosec®, antacids, like TUMS®, laxatives, antispasmodics, or antidepressants. Soon enough, you discovered you were right back where you started and that your digestive system seemed out of whack again! This can be very frustrating. The good news is that you don't have to continue this vicious cycle. There are proactive things you can do to help permanently improve your digestive system! Here are **5 great soothing GI tips** that you may not have heard or thought of! Go ahead and try them; you may surprise yourself!

Soothing Tip #1: Soluble Fiber

Foods that are high in soluble fiber include: rice, oatmeal, barley, soy, applesauce, carrots, beets, avocados, squash and bananas. Soluble fiber attracts water and creates a gel-like consistency in the gut. This material helps to slow down digestion and can make you feel full. What a bonus for weight loss! In addition, soluble fiber can help regulate blood sugar levels, leading to improved insulin secretion.

Soothing Tip #2: Power of Peppermint!

There is nothing like having a cup of peppermint tea right after a good meal! Peppermint has been known for its ability to relieve gas and bloating. Peppermint relaxes the smooth muscles in the digestive tract, promoting a sense of comfort and good digestive breakdown. It is mostly known for its antispasmodic properties. If you have reflux, be cautious with excess peppermint intake, as it can have a relaxing effect on the lower esophageal sphincter and exacerbate this issue.

Soothing Tip #3: Lady Fingers?

Did you know that okra is known as lady fingers? This plant belongs to the "Mallow" family and is known for its mucilaginous consistency. This slippery texture aids in digestion by promoting peristalsis by absorbing water and bulking up stool. In addition, the mucilage action coats and lubricates the digestive tract, providing a protective barrier. The fiber in okra is beneficial at promoting probiotic activity in the intestines.

Ever Tried Yoga?

If not, now can be the time to learn a few cool moves that will help your intestinal tract function. Triangle pose is known as Trikonasana in Sanskrit - tri meaning three and kona meaning corner - and it helps to improve digestive aliments.

Soothing Tip #4: Triangle Pose

Have you ever tried yoga? If not, now can be the time to learn a few cool moves that will help your intestinal tract function. Triangle pose is known as Trikonasana in Sanskrit—tri meaning three and kona meaning corner - and it helps to improve digestive aliments. Triangle pose consists of stretching the abdominal muscles, neck, back and legs. This pose helps to increase bowel activity by promoting movement of food content through the intestines, thereby alleviating constipation.

Soothing Tip #5: Cardamom – Queen of Spices!

The King of Spices is known as black pepper, and the Queen is known as cardamom! Ancient Egyptians and Greeks used Cardamom to help with dental disease, bad breath and digestive complaints. This aromatic and ginger-like plant has a pungent and warm taste is carminative in nature, and is underused in our diet today. It is an excellent remedy for flatulence, upset stomach, and abdominal pain.

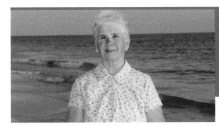

Healthy Brain & Memory Boosters

By Dr. Adrienne Stewart

There are several things you can do to strengthen your memory so that it does not fade with age. Incorporating these healthy techniques into your daily life can keep your mind sharp. These techniques improve many areas of cognitive function, including concentration, mood, short-term memory, and mental clarity.

Exercise for a Healthy Brain

A great way to improve brain function is to increase blood circulation. Blood carries nutrients and oxygen needed to keep brain tissue healthy. To increase blood flow, increasing activity is what matters most. Be sure to give yourself hourly movement and stretching breaks. A great way to increase your exercise routine is to choose activities that are cheerful, challenging, and consistent.

You can also enhance blood flow through breathing exercises, such as alternate nostril breathing. To do this, gently close one nostril with one finger while breathing deeply from the other nostril. After a deep breath, you switch nostrils by gently closing the other and breathing deeply. Not only does this exercise improve blood circulation, it's been shown to improve spatial memory. Another effective way to "exercise" the brain is to routinely engage both sides of the brain with music, art, reading, and games such as crossword puzzles and Sudoku.

Lifestyle for a Healthy Brain

Stress and poor sleep can take a toll on brain health over time. Chronic stress can spike certain chemicals in the brain that disrupt sleep cycles. Practices such as mindful meditation and yoga can help reduce stress and improve sleep. Good sleep hygiene is also essential, and includes a relaxing bedtime routine, a dark and quiet room, and at least 8 hours of high-quality sleep with few interruptions. Avoid television and computers at least an hour before bed because of how the light effects your sleep cycles. Other sleep disruptors include alcohol and caffeine. Avoiding them, and cigarette smoke, is essential for a healthy brain. Another brain boost is a diet full of antioxidants in the form of berries, dark green vegetables, beans, legumes, and green tea. Antioxidants help repair and protect brain tissue from oxidative stress. Another way to feed your brain is with an anti-inflammatory diet rich in essential fatty acids like EPA and DHA. These healthy fats can be found in food sources such as wild salmon, sardines, flax, walnuts, and grassfed meats.

Supplements for a Healthy Brain

Adding in supplements can give your brain the extra boost it needs for optimal performance. Herbs like Ginkgo biloba and Bacopa can help with brain cognition and memory recall by increasing blood flow and providing neuroprotective and antioxidant properties. Nutrients such as Acetyl-L-Carnitine and Phosphatidylserine are essential for optimal brain function. Both have been shown in research studies to improve memory and cognitive performance. Vinpocetine, a nutrient derived from the Periwinkle plant, is another helpful nutrient for cerebral circulation and oxygen utilization.

Hidden Obstacles for Healthy Brains

Some symptoms of cognitive difficulties, like foggy thinking, can actually be signs of heavy metal toxicity, not aging. Toxin avoidance and detoxing from heavy metals can dramatically improve brain health.

Another commonly overlooked area is hormonal imbalances. This can range from low thyroid, adrenal stress imbalances, or low estrogen levels.

Remember that you do not have to walk your journey alone. One of the most important aspects of health is having a loving system of support from family, friends, and health professionals who care.

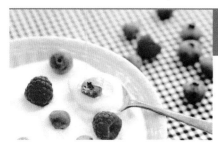

Probiotics

By Dr. Alan Christianson

Did you know that you are composed of 1000 times more bacteria than human cells? Hundreds of different species of bacteria live in every nook and cranny of your body – inside and out.

What was once thought to be a bunch of freeloaders now is known to be as important as your liver or kidneys. You serve as their host, almost like a cruise liner for them. It is in their interest for the ship to not sink. Consequently, these bacteria work together in complex ways to regulate your body's chemistry.

They do this by communicating with one another by releasing small chemical messengers. These messengers can be thought of as similar to the pheromones released by moths and butterflies. By the number and types of chemical messengers in circulation, bacteria 'know' how large the colony is of each species and how healthy each colony is. They are able to adjust their activity and their individual numbers in ways that benefit your body.

Do you remember the Flinstones' cartoons? One of the historical inaccuracies was that prehistoric humans did not have refrigeration. In fact, scientists believe that our ancestors consumed significant amounts of decomposing food. As long as it wasn't too ripe, they would have been given high doses of bacteria, most of which were helpful. This is how we came to be dependent on bacteria.

Bacteria Helps Maintain Your Health
The main roles they help us with include:

Regulation of your immune system

Formation of nutrients from foods

Controlling how you eliminate your hormones

Breaking down chemical toxins from your body

Effecting how you read your genetic code

Studies have shown that these roles have specific and measurable effects on your health. Types and amounts of good bacteria have been shown to influence numerous diseases, including:

Obesity	Chronic Fatigue	Stroke	Acne
Ulcerative Colitis	Eczema	Fibromyalgia	Arthritis
Kidney disease	Bladder infections	Psoriasis	Crohn's Disease

Balance of Healthy Bacteria Key to Health
Given the importance of good bacteria, it is apparent that keeping them healthy will keep you healthy. They work like a compost pile, breaking down wastes to make healthy soil. If the wrong things go into the compost, you get mold instead of healthy soil.

Likewise, our good bacteria are vulnerable to going wrong. The term 'dysbiosis,' refers to any state of our bacteria that works against our health. Unfortunately, many factors common to modern life can hurt our good bacteria. These include:

Processed Sugar	Oral Antibiotics	Oral Contraceptives	Chlorinated Water
Fluoridated Water	Pesticides from Food	Hand Sanitizers	Food Preservatives
Stress	Low Fiber Diets	Prescription Medicines	Excess Alcohol

It is apparent how valuable and how vulnerable our bacteria are. Keeping them working for us is a worthwhile effort.

How to Make Your Bacteria Work for You

Step 1
Avoid all the above factors that hurt them. Eating organic, minimally processed foods is the best way to do this. Never fear washing with soap but do avoid frequent use of hand sanitizers and products with antimicrobial chemicals.

Step 2
Include naturally fermented foods in your diet. This DOES NOT include the four-day-old potato salad left over from the family picnic. The easiest versions to start with include:
- Miso
- Kimchee
- Sauerkraut

Miso is a brown paste which is made into a broth. Most have soy, but many soy-free versions are available. My favorite recipe for miso soup is pretty simple. Slice a green onion into small pieces. Add it and 1 Tbs. of miso to a cup of hot water. Mix well, let sit for 3 minutes and enjoy.

Kimchee is a wonderful traditional Korean food. Like sauerkraut, it is fermented cabbage. Unlike sauerkraut, it is very flavorful. It is made with lots of garlic and chilies. A tablespoon or so works great alongside most meals.

Good Bacteria

Include naturally fermented foods in your diet, such as miso, kimchee or sauerkraut. Supplements can also be taken in the form of pills, drinks or chewables.

Most people have had sauerkraut. It is a great food that goes well with any protein dish. Keep the quantities under a cup to avoid excess sodium.

All of these foods can be found at health food supermarkets. Look for raw, unpasteurized versions.

Step 3
Good bacteria can also be supplemented. Many supplements that contain them are available in pills, drinks, and chewable. Unfortunately, they are hard to keep stable after production. Probiotic supplements do not have any known side effects or harmful interactions with drugs. Some people who really lack their own good flora may notice gas or looser stools the first few days they use probiotics. This does pass, no pun intended!

When independent assays are done, most products are found to have few viable bacteria remaining. Refrigerated products are not more apt to be stable than non-refrigerated.

Among products with good quality control, the strongest predictor of how well they will work is quite simply the number of viable bacteria available. The more good bacteria you get per serving, the more they can help your health.

Products have really gotten better in the recent past. The best products used to have 500 million bacteria. Then many came out with 10-20 billion. My current favorite has 225 billion good bacteria of many different strains. This is so powerful that you can take 1 dose weekly for maintenance. Those with immune or digestive problems can take a daily dose for 1 month, then go on to weekly dosing.

Assuming you are not planning on eating decomposing food, probiotics are worth supplementing regularly. Benefits can include better skin, less bloating and easier weight loss.

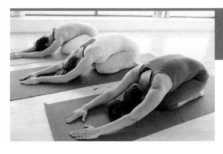

Yoga for Apnea?

By Dr. Alan Christianson

Are you more tired than you should be? Do you get edgy too easily? Are you prone to headaches in the morning?

Something you may not have thought to be a possible culprit is sleep apnea. We suspect this with the above symptoms. This is more suspicious when someone is known to snore, have trouble staying asleep, or breathe erratically at night.

Here's a quirky hint that you might have apnea: your dreams may be clues. Even though we are asleep, our brain retains some awareness of our body's experience as we dream. Oftentimes these experiences are translated into our dreams. Ever dream of trying to find a bathroom before waking up and using one for real? This is a great example.

Dreams of flying, dreams of being underwater, dreams of smoking or breathing through a straw can all be common signs of apnea.

Apnea is a big deal. It raises the risk for stroke, dementia and heart attacks. Oh yeah – it can also cause weight gain.

Classic apnea sufferers are male, overweight, alcohol users and stressed. Yet younger, lean, non-drinking females can still have it.

Many who have suspected apnea have been resistant to do anything about it for fear of having to struggle with the breathing devices called CPAP machines. Since apnea is related to muscular weakness of the throat, many suspected that exercises could help with it without the need to sleep in a diving apparatus.

Several large studies have shown that this can work. Some involved detailed specific exercises, some involved normal training in musical wind instruments. One showed that playing the Didgeridoo can work also, though the loincloth is optional. If you have suspected apnea, take it seriously. Those who suffer from it report life-changing benefits when it improves.

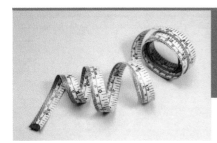

Acupuncture for Weight Loss

By Dr. Linda Khoshaba

Acupuncture for weight loss is a great way to jump-start and reset your metabolism. This form of Traditional Chinese Medicine has been used for thousands of years and has been shown to help with numerous health conditions. Acupuncture for weight loss has been used to stimulate the pituitary gland, also known as the master gland, because it controls endocrine hormones. These hormones are responsible for sending a signal to your brain to reduce cravings, increase energy, and reset hormones that influence the eating response. Two hormones in particular, Ghrelin and Leptin, have a direct effect on metabolism. Ghrelin is a hormone that is responsible for increasing your appetite and Leptin is the one responsible for suppressing it. An easy way to remember the functions of these is to think of Ghrelin as the one that makes your stomach growl and Leptin is the one responsible for making you eat less. Acupuncture is a powerful, safe, and natural alternative that can help to balance the ratio between these hormones, and many others in the body.

Acupuncture works on the body's total energy system, with different points on the body representing specific functions. Acupuncture for weight loss has a variety of points, particularly located on the ear. The ear itself is a micro-representation of the entire body, as it is shaped like an inverted fetus. There are different anatomical points used for many conditions. Acupuncture to lose weight includes using four main auricular points: Hunger Point, Endocrine Point, Shen Men (aka Heavenly Gate), and the Stomach Point. When used in combination with each other, there is a reset in homeostasis balancing energy, emotions and hormones.

If you are considering acupuncture to lose weight, there are a few things to keep in mind. First of all, it is important to understand that acupuncture works in conjunction with a good diet and exercise program. It is not a replacement for lifestyle factors, but can work to increase energy that will improve weight loss. In addition, acupuncture is not usually a one-time treatment. In order to achieve optimal results for any health condition, a series of acupuncture treatments over the course of a couple of months is usually adequate. When considering an acupuncturist, make sure you find someone who is qualified, as this can vary state to state. In some states, a medical doctor can perform acupuncture for weight loss. In other states, a person that has attained a Master's degree in acupuncture is also qualified.

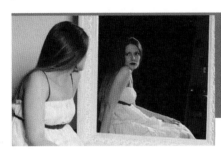

Stop Checking Yourself Out in the Mirror

By Dr. Alan Christianson

You incorporate protein at every meal, provide your body optimal nutrients, combine burst training with weight resistance four times each week, and turned down numerous late-night dates with your girlfriends to meet your eight-hour nightly sleep quota.

Your herculean efforts have paid off. You're finally able to get into those Size 4 skinny jeans for your best friend's much-anticipated dinner party this Saturday night.

Looking hot is its own reward. But when you lose weight, you gain numerous health benefits that go way beyond vanity.

Here are seven post-weight loss benefits you might not consider because you're too busy checking out your sexy, lean figure in the mirror.

1. Live longer.
Burn fat and you have a better chance of enjoying and thriving during your twilight years. A 14-year study in *The New England Journal of Medicine* with

1.46 million adults concluded mortality is lowest when you keep your Body Mass Index (BMI) within the normal range of 20 – 24.9.

A healthy weight means you're less prone to diseases that steal decades from your life.

For instance, this study found obese participants (with a BMI over 30) had a 40 – 80 percent higher risk of dying from cancer than normal-weight people. Heart disease also skyrockets; obese men here were three times more likely to die from heart disease than normal-weight males.

Live Longer!

A healthy weight means you're less prone to diseases that steal decades from your life.

Living longer means nothing, however, if you can't enjoy that time. Fortunately, your quality of life also improves when you lose weight.

A study in *Obesity Research* found that the more weight you lose, the better quality of life measures you have, such as physical function, self-esteem, and sex life.

2. Alleviate arthritis.
Excess weight increases stress on your knees, triggering cartilage breakdown and eventually, arthritis. Overweight women are four times more likely to develop knee arthritis. For overweight men, that risk becomes five times higher.

Even losing a small amount of weight can reduce your risk for arthritis. And if you already have arthritis, losing fat can reduce pain and cartilage breakdown.

In the famous Framingham Study, for instance, for every 11 pounds women lost, knee arthritis risk dropped about 50%. (The converse also occurred: women who gained weight increased their risk of later developing knee arthritis.)

And don't think your other joints are off the hook: studies show excess weight can exacerbate arthritis throughout your body.

A study in the *American Journal of Preventive Medicine* found a strong relationship between body weight and arthritis. Maintaining a healthy weight, they concluded, can delay the onset of arthritis.

3. Reduce your risk for diabetes.

Obesity is the major risk factor for type 2 diabetes, and about 80 – 90% of people with diabetes have a BMI above 30.

A study in the *American Journal of Medicine* with 21,000 men found that elevated BMI hugely influences your risk for diabetes, although physical activity can somewhat reduce that risk.

The highly processed carbs/low-fiber American diet practically invites type 2 diabetes.

Your hormone insulin's job is to remove sugar from your blood and get it into your cells, which use it for energy. The higher your blood sugar, the more insulin your pancreas produces.

> ### Did you know?
>
> *The highly processed carbs/low-fiber American diet practically invites type 2 diabetes.*

Insulin does one thing *really* well: it stores fat. Eventually, your cells get burned out, and insulin resistance (the beginning of diabetes) occurs.

A study at the National Institutes for Health shows being at a healthy weight reduces your risk for type 2 diabetes up to 70 percent. The good news: Every pound you lose improves your health.

Of course, when you lose weight, you also reduce or eliminate the numerous complications of diabetes, which include hypoglycemia, atherosclerosis, neuropathy, immune system dysfunction, depression, and cognitive issues.

4. Reduce inflammation.

Doctors have called inflammation the silent killer and connected this condition with every degenerative disease from cancer to cognitive decline to, yes, obesity. A vicious cycle ensues: obesity triggers inflammation, which in turn makes you fatter.

There are two varieties of inflammation. When you cut your finger, acute inflammation signals white blood cells to the area. You *want* this kind of inflammation. Otherwise, you'd bleed to death. But sometimes inflammation goes into overdrive and lingers around far longer than your body needs it. Rather than protect, it begins to damage your body.

Chronic inflammation could explain why overweight people are more susceptible to heart disease, cancer, and other illnesses.

Losing weight reduces inflammation. For instance, a study in the *American Journal of Clinical Nutrition* found that weight loss reduces overall inflammation in older, obese persons. And a study in the journal *Clinical Science* found weight loss was the primary factor to significantly reduce inflammatory markers.

Besides weight loss itself, the right kind of diet can reduce inflammation. The American diet is high in pro-inflammatory foods like wheat and vegetable oils. When you shift to fat-burning, anti-inflammatory foods like fresh fruit and vegetables, as well omega-3 fatty acids, you also help combat inflammation.

5. Have better sex.

Weight loss might be the spark that reignites your passion. When you're lean, your partner finds you more attractive and you feel more confident. That confidence spills over to the bedroom.

Have better sex

A study in the journal Obesity found almost 30 percent of obese people have reduced levels of sex drive, desire, and/or performance.

Being overweight can have the opposite effect on your sex drive. A study in the journal *Obesity* found almost 30 percent of obese people have reduced levels of sex drive, desire, and/or performance.

Researchers found that insulin resistance and other obesity-related conditions, for instance, restrict the tiny arteries that distribute blood to the genitals.

Being overweight will also age you sexually. A study in the *Journal of the American College of Surgeons* found that middle-aged morbidly obese men have sexual dysfunction issues equivalent to normal-weight men 20 years older. Not surprisingly, their sexual health vastly improved when they lost weight.

A fat-burning diet rich in wild salmon and other seafood, green leafy vegetables, berries, and even indulgent foods in moderation, like dark chocolate and red wine, can boost your libido and balance your blood sugar so you don't have the fatigue and other problems that zap your sex drive.

6. Better mental function.

Being lean reduces your risk factors for brain diseases like Alzheimer's, sleep apnea, and stroke. A study in the journal *Surgery for Obesity and Related Diseases* found that losing weight could also improve cognitive function.

Researchers measured memory and attention levels in 150 overweight participants who completed mental-skills tests to determine their recall and attention at the beginning of the study and again 12 weeks later after they lost weight.

When the study began, about 24 percent of the patients showed impaired learning and 23 percent showed signs of poor memory recall when tested.

By the end of the study, participants had lost an average of 17 percent of their initial body weight and boosted their scores into average or above-average cognitive range.

Researchers concluded that being overweight impacts metabolic pathways that affect how your brain processes information. Becoming lean provides the spark plug to boost cognition.

7. Better mood.

When you lose weight, you increase self-esteem levels. You feel great about your body and that infectious confidence shows.

Because you're eating healthier, you're not sending your blood sugar on a roller coaster ride that leaves you crashing mid-morning, suffering lethargy and brain fog, and snapping at a coworker.

Get happy

When you lose weight, you increase self-esteem levels. You feel great about your body and that infectious confidence shows.

A study in *The American Journal of Clinical Nutrition* concluded a high-protein breakfast reduces your levels of ghrelin, the hormone that tells your brain to eat now, much better than a carb-heavy breakfast.

When ghrelin levels stay elevated, you're hungry, tired, cranky, and hardly enthusiastic about the day ahead.

But when you start your day with a protein-based meal such as a smoothie loaded with berries, fiber, a quality protein power and coconut milk, you have steady, sustained energy, which means you stay full, focused, and feeling amazing all morning.

So now when you do check yourself out in the mirror, remember to give yourself kudos for all the hidden benefits you've gained from losing the weight.

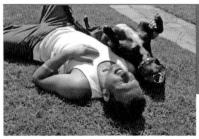

7 Step Worksheet to a Healthy Weight

By Dr. Adrienne Stewart

1. Find Your Purpose For Losing Weight

Beyond making a goal, what brings you joy? Is there someone that can help support you or can you support someone else to lose the weight?

My purpose for losing weight is

_____.

2. Be Mindful of What & How You Eat

Eliminate the junk (sodas, sugar, processed foods) and watch portion sizes. Consider keeping a diet diary. How mindful are you when you eat?

One change that I can make immediately is

_____.

3. Make Exercise Fun

Block time for exercise and make your health a priority.
What are some aerobic and anaerobic exercises you enjoy doing?
Find an exercise partner or a fun group class.

One exercise challenge I am setting for myself this year is

_____.

4. Manage Your Stress, Don't Let Stress Manage You

Cortisol is a stress hormone that promotes weight gain, especially in the abdominal area. Some strategies include meditation, yoga, journaling, and deep breathing techniques.

One strategy for stress management that I can do is

_____.

5. Eat Breakfast
It is important to have stable blood sugar throughout the day. Protein options include eggs (if you are not allergic) and rice and pea protein powders. A nutritious and protein-rich breakfast that I will start incorporating into my diet includes

_____.

6. Reduce Your Toxin Burden
The best detox is to first practice avoidance. Stopping smoking, drinking, or other recreational drugs can make a huge impact on your weight. Another quick start is to avoid the EWG's Dirty Dozen™ and eat the Clean 15™ foods.

I can reduce my toxin exposure by

_____.

7. Eliminate Your Individual Food Sensitivities
With a simple blood test, we can test for food allergies and sensitivities. You may also consider an elimination diet of some of the most common sensitivities, including dairy, gluten, eggs, corn, soy, peanuts, sugar and artificial sweeteners.

One step that I can take to help manage my food sensitivities is

_____.

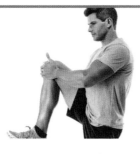

What is Prolotherapy?

Prolotherapy, *which comes from the word "proliferate,"* is a method of injection treatment designed to stimulate healing of injured ligaments and tendons. Various irritant solutions are injected into the ligaments, tendons and joints to encourage repair of damaged tissue. Strengthening disabled ligaments and tendons by stimulating the wound healing process is how prolotherapy works. Macrophages, a type of white blood cells, activate wound healing and initiate growth and proliferation.

Wound healing involves **3 distinct phases** that overlap:
1. Inflammation 2. Granulation 3. Remodeling.

BENEFITS OF PROLOTHERAPY:

Naturally relieves pain permanently

Improves stability and function!

Safe and effective!

Simulates body's wound healing process to regenerate collagen

More effective than corticosteroid injections!

Strengthens ligaments and tendons

What should I expect from Prolotherapy?

After your procedure, we encourage activity to stress the lines of force through the tissue. We highly recommend you avoid NSAIDs for 4 days pre- and post-injection. If you require some pain relief, analgesics for pain (usually narcotics for the first 3-5 days) are preferred. We recommend 3-6 sessions at 3-4 week intervals.

Common Problems that Respond to Prolotherapy

Joint instability: Ankle, knee, hip, sacroiliac, shoulder, wrist and digits

Fibromyalgia, i.e. tendonosis

Spinal pain due to tendonosis or ligament laxity

Persistent post-MVA pain, occipital headaches

Piriformis syndrome

What Causes Ligament Laxity?

Incomplete wound healing

Recurrent trauma (overuse injuries)

Overwhelming tissue trauma

Hormonal deficiencies: thyroid, estrogen, testosterone or hGh

Nutritional deficiencies

What are some signs of Ligament Laxity?

Pain – local/referred

Joint hypermobility/spasm of associated muscles

Trigger points in associated muscles

Weakness/atrophy of associated muscles

Somatic dysfunction and morning stiffness

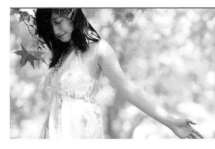

Nutrient IVs & Booster Shots

Need a quick boost? It's no secret that nutrients make us feel good. It's also no secret that they take a lot of time and work to get into our bodies. Many nutrients can also be hard to absorb even if we get them in pills or foods. The advantage is that an IV can bypass the gastrointestinal system where many nutrients may get "lost" due to a poor digestive system. In addition, higher amounts of certain nutrients can be administered to promote a healthy, safe, and fast therapeutic effect.

Since 1996, we have made custom blends of nutrients to help our patients feel their best. Due to popular demand, we've made a menu of some of our best formulas.

Nutrient IVs

Super Immune

Stop your cold, flu or bronchitis in its tracks	Reduce body aches
	Break the cycle of repeated infections
Restore lost electrolytes	Prevent seasonal sinus infections
Relax constricted lungs	Travel without fear of getting ill
Eliminate phlegm and mucus	

Usage tips: Get in for a Super Immune IV when the very first symptoms show up. To make this IV work even better, take a hot bath at night before bed, wrap up in extra blankets and get plenty of rest. The Super Immune IV is popular before a major trip or before attending events with exposure to large crowds.

Energy & Nutrient Support

Give yourself an energy boost when feeling run down or before a special event

Make up for the supplements you forget to take

Help promote growth of muscle tissue

Encourage growth of healthy bones

Resolve chronic anemias

Cure painful muscle cramps

Usage tips: Do you hate taking supplements? Or at times, do you just forget? You're not alone – an Energy & Nutrient Support IV may be the solution for you!

Everyday Detox

Stimulate the growth of new liver cells

Eliminate years of stored toxins

Improve quality of skin

Decrease painful headaches

Usage tips: If you're feeling bloated or toxic, this is the IV for you. You can't live without your liver. Do you have any idea how hard it has to work every day to detox your blood? Do it a favor and detox it for a change!

Pre/Post-Surgery

Eliminate residue of general anesthesia

Regain brain function

Speed rate of healing

Lower risk of permanent scars

Strengthen immunity to lower risk of post-surgical infection

Maximize nerve regeneration

Usage tips: Great to do in the days before and immediately after surgery. This IV is designed to build tissue integrity and help you heal.

Serenity

Reduce anxiety

Overcome stress from work or hectic daily schedules

Increase a sense of calmness

Usage tips: Great to do when you need to take some time for yourself and lie back in one of our zerogravity recliners.

Hydration

Reverse dehydration, especially from vomiting or diarrhea

Hydrate all your cells – including your skin

Usage tips: Be sure to drink lots of water with electrolytes. Great to do when nothing seems to be quenching your thirst, and during the hot summer months.

Other Prescription IVs Our Clinic Offers

Heavy Metal Detox	Asthma & Lung Support
Heart Health Chelation	Blood Pressure Support
High Dose Vitamin C	Amino Acid Booster
ALA Nerve Support	Plus Custom IVs
Joint Pain Relief	

Booster IM Shots

Our anytime booster shots have got you covered! Whether it's an immune, energy or serenity boost, you will be feeling your best with our custom IM shots.

Booster IM Shots
Looking for a quick and efficient boost? Our anytime booster shots have got you covered! Whether it's an immune, energy or serenity boost, you will be feeling your best with our custom IM shots.

B-12 Bomber
Sure to rev up your engine with many days of heightened energy and no crash.

Ultimate B:
For the most in energy, mental focus and physical stamina. Includes B-12 + B Complex + Folic Acid

Super Antioxidant:
A super boost of glutathione, the body's most powerful antioxidant. Perfect antidote for stress, alcohol and modern life in general.

Immunity Booster:
Stimulate your own body's immune system with this quick homeopathic shot.

Liquid Serenity:
Magnesium sulfate naturally relaxes muscles and soothes anxiety. Perfect to help restore sleep and ease tension.

Lipo-Dissolve:
Stimulate your metabolism to get to your ideal level of leanness.

AMP:
Adenosine monophosphate is what your cells work so hard to make to release energy. Now you can have more of it in a pure state. Natural energy burst for days, no crash of jitters.

Anti-Nausea:
Feeling the effects of pregnancy, or just want to feel better in a pinch? Our anti-nausea will soothe your tummy and GI tract.

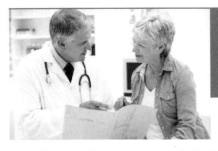

Understanding Your Blood Test

You and your doctor can tell a great deal about your health by testing a sample of your blood. Laboratory tests help in several ways. Sometimes test results will be abnormal before you have any symptoms, and when you have symptoms, laboratory test results help confirm that a problem does exist.

A normal test result is just as significant as an abnormal result. A normal result does not mean that the test was unnecessary. When a result is normal, it not only helps to rule out disease, but it also establishes a baseline "normal." A person's own normal result is the best baseline for monitoring any change that takes place in the future.

What follows is a brief description of the typical tests that may be included in a testing profile. These descriptions will help you to better understand your laboratory test results so that you may have a more meaningful discussion with your doctor. You should not rely on this information for diagnostic treatment. These descriptions are not intended to be a complete listing of all conditions medically relevant to each test. Always consult your doctor regarding your laboratory tests.

Glucose
Glucose is the chief source of energy for all living organisms; however, abnormally high or low blood glucose levels may be a sign of disease. For example, high glucose levels after 12 hours of fasting may suggest diabetes. Low blood glucose, on the other hand, may be seen with certain tumors or with liver disease. A low glucose level may also mean that the blood sample was not handled property after it was drawn.

Uric Acid
Uric acid levels are useful in the diagnosis of gout. Gout is a condition that occurs and affects men more than women. Diets high in purines (present in sweetbreads, kidney, and liver) may worsen the condition. Patients with gout may develop arthritis and/or kidney stones. A number of drugs, particularly diuretics and salicylates (aspirin), may also increase uric acid. Uric acid levels may be increased during kidney failure, with certain tumors, and as a response to stress and alcohol.

Phosphate

Phosphate is closely associated with calcium in bone development and is primarily found in the bones. The remaining phosphate level, which is found in the blood, is very important for muscle and nerve function. Very low levels of phosphate in the blood can be associated with starvation or malnutrition and this can lead to muscle weakness. High levels of phosphate in the blood are usually associated with kidney disease.

Calcium

Calcium is one of the most important elements in the body. Ninety-nine percent of the calcium in the body is in the bones. The remaining one percent is in body fluids, such as nerves, enzymes, muscles, and blood clotting. High levels can be caused by bone disease, excess intake of antacids and milk (this is often seen in people with ulcers), excessive intake of vitamin D, and overactivity of the thyroid gland. The parathyroid gland is the main regulator of calcium in the body. Tumors of the parathyroid gland may result in very high calcium levels.

> ## Calcium
>
> *Calcium is one of the most important elements in the body. Ninety-nine percent of the calcium in the body is in the bones.*

Magnesium

This element is found primarily inside the cells of the body. Like calcium, the level in the blood is important. A low magnesium level in the blood may indicate severe malnutrition, severe diarrhea, alcoholism, or excessive use of diuretics. A very low level of magnesium in the blood can cause your muscles to tremble.

Total Bilirubin

Bilirubin is the pigment in the blood that makes your blood plasma or serum yellow. When the bilirubin level in the blood is very high, the whites of your eyes and your skin may become yellow. This is known as jaundice. Bilirubin comes from the breakdown of old red cells in the blood. A high bilirubin level in the blood can be caused by too many red cells being destroyed (hemolysis), by liver disease, or by a blockage of the bile ducts. Fasting can also cause a slight increase in total bilirubin.

Direct Bilirubin

This is a specific form of bilirubin that is formed in the liver and excreted in the bile. Normally, very little of this form of bilirubin is present in the blood, so even a slightly high level of direct bilirubin indicates a problem with the liver cells.

Alkaline Phosphatase

Alkaline Phosphatase is found in all body tissue, but the most important sites are bone and liver. Blood levels increase when bones are growing, thus children have higher levels than adults do. High levels may also be seen in bone and liver disease. Certain drugs may cause high levels, too.

Gamma-Glutamyl Transferase (GGT)

GGT is primarily found in the liver. Drinking too much alcohol, certain drugs, obstructive liver disease, and bile duct disease can cause high levels of GGT in the blood.

Aspartate Aminotransferase (AST)

AST is found mainly in the heart, liver, and muscles. High levels of AST in the blood suggest a problem with the heart, liver, or muscles.

Lactate Dehydrogenase (LDH)

LDH is found in all tissues in the body, thus a high level in the blood can result from a number of different diseases. Slightly elevated levels In the blood are common and rarely indicate disease. The most common sources of LDH are the heart, liver, muscles, and red blood cells.

Blood Urea Nitrogen (BUN)

BUN is a waste product derived from protein breakdown in the liver and excreted by the kidneys. When your kidneys are not working well, the level of BUN in the blood will rise. Dehydration and blood loss can also cause a high BUN level. Liver disease, a low protein diet, or too much water intake may cause a low BUN level.

Creatinine

The blood concentration of creatinine depends upon two things – the amount of muscle you have and the ability of your kidneys to excrete the creatinine. A high level of creatinine in the blood usually indicates deterioration in the kidney function.

BUN/Creatinine Ratio

When BUN and/or creatinine levels are abnormal, the doctor can determine if the high BUN level is caused by a kidney problem or from something like blood loss in the abdomen.

Albumin

Approximately two-thirds of the total protein circulating in your blood is albumin. This important protein keeps water inside your blood vessels. When your albumin level is too low, water can leak out of your blood vessels into other parts of your body and cause swelling. A low level of albumin in the blood can be caused by malnutrition, too much water in the body, liver disease, kidney disease, severe injury such as burns or major bone fractures, and slow bleeding over a long period of time.

Globulin

This is the group of proteins in your blood that helps to fight infections. It is actually comprised of about 60 different important proteins. Some of the proteins in the group play an important role in blood clotting. If your globulin level is abnormal, your doctor may want to measure some of the individual proteins that make up this group.

Albumin/Globulin Ratio

A simple way to tell if the albumin or globulin levels in the blood are abnormal is to compare the level of albumin to the level of globulin in your blood.

Sodium

This element plays an important role in salt and water balance in your body. The adrenal hormone, aldosterone, and the rate of excretion in urine, regulate the blood sodium level. Too much water intake, heart failure, or kidney failure because of fluid retention can cause a low sodium level in the blood. A low level can also be caused by loss of sodium in diarrhea, fluid , and vomit, or by a deficiency of adrenal hormone. Too much intake of salt or not enough intake of water can cause a high level.

Sodium

This element plays an important role in salt and water balance in your body.

Potassium

This element is found inside all cells. Its role is to maintain water balance inside the cells and help in the transmission of nerve impulses. The level of potassium in blood is of critical significance. Low levels may be found in patients on diuretics or in patients not receiving enough dietary potassium. A low potassium level can cause muscle weakness and heart problems. A high level can be found in kidney disease or in overuse of potassium supplements. Some "salt" substitutes contain potassium instead of sodium, and an excessive use of these substitutes can cause dangerously high levels of potassium in the blood. Adrenal hormone disorders can also alter blood potassium levels.

Chloride

Chloride is another element that plays a role in salt and water balance. It is almost never the only element that is low or high. Changes in the chloride level are usually associated with changes in sodium or potassium. Borderline low or high levels of chloride usually have very little significance. When there is too much or too little acid in the blood, chloride is an important clue to the cause of the acid abnormality.

Iron

The body must have iron to make hemoglobin and to help transfer oxygen to the muscles.

Iron

The body must have iron to make hemoglobin and to help transfer oxygen to the muscles. If the body is low in iron, all body cells, particularly muscles in adults and brain cells in children, do not function properly. On the other hand, if there is too much iron in the body, this can cause injury to the heart, pancreas, joints, testicles, ovaries, etc. Iron excess is found in the heredity disease called hemochromatosis, which can be found in about 3 out of every 1000 people.

Total Iron Binding Capacity (TIBC)

Iron is transported in your blood bound to a protein called transferin. Transferin transports the iron in your body from the iron storage sites to where it is needed. It also transports the iron, when not needed back to the storage sites. A low TIBC suggests malnutrition or iron excess. A high TIBC suggests iron deficiency.

Transferin Percent Saturation

This percent is obtained by comparing the iron level to the TIBC level. It is a simple way to compare the amount of iron in the blood to the capacity of the blood to transport iron.

Cholesterol

Cholesterol is an essential blood fat, but too high a level of this fat is associated with a higher risk of heart disease and clogged blood vessels. The total cholesterol level in blood includes LDL (bad cholesterol) and HDL (good cholesterol).

HDL Cholesterol

High-density lipoprotein (HDL) cholesterol is sometimes described as the "good" cholesterol. One of the important roles of HDL cholesterol in your body is to carry cholesterol away from your arteries to your liver. The more HDL cholesterol you have, the more cholesterol can be carried away and not clog your arteries.

Cholesterol/ HDL Cholesterol Ratio

This number is obtained by comparing the total cholesterol level to the HDL cholesterol level. The higher the number, the greater the risk of coronary heart disease. A high HDL cholesterol level will result in a lower ratio, which means a lower risk. This could be true even if the total cholesterol level is high.

Triglycerides
This is a blood fat largely derived from dietary fat absorption and, to a limited extent, related to higher risk of heart disease. You must not eat for at least 12 hours to obtain an accurate result for this test.

High-Sensitivity CRP
CRP (C-Reactive Protein) is a protein produced in the liver that circulates in the blood. High-Sensitivity CRP is a blood test that is able to detect small amounts of CRP. Even low levels of CRP can help indicate your risk for heart disease and help predict risk of a first heart attack up to eight years in advance.

Triglycerides
This is a blood fat largely derived from dietary fat absorption and, to a limited extent, related to higher risk of heart disease.

TSH (Thyroid Stimulating Hormone)
When your TSH is above normal, it means you have too small an amount of thyroid hormones, and in response your pituitary gland is releasing more TSH than usual to tell your thyroid to step up production. Conversely, if your TSH is below normal, it means you have too great an amount of thyroid hormones, an in response your pituitary gland is releasing less TSH than usual to slow your thyroid's production. In other words, there's an inverse relationship between your TSH and thyroid hormone levels because your pituitary gland is continually trying to address any imbalance.

Free T4 and Free T3
Thyroid hormones control the rate at which energy is used and released by the body. A low level of thyroid hormones (hypothyroidism) may cause tiredness, depression, or weight gain. A high level of thyroid hormones (hyperthyroidism) may cause nervousness, irritability or weight loss. Unlike the TSH test which reflects a 2-3 month average, the free T4 and free T3 tests reflect the activities of those hormones within the past 7-14 days. Evaluating your TSH level in conjunction with free T4 and free T3 levels provides a much clearer view of your thyroid hormone balance.

Thyroglobulin Antibody (TgAb) and Thyroid Peroxidase Antibody (TPOAb)
These tests help diagnose and monitor Hashimoto's Thyroiditis, which is an autoimmune thyroid disease. They also help us guide treatment decisions for optimal thyroid balance.

Cortisol

Blood cortisol testing is used to help screen for and diagnose adrenal diseases, such as Cushing's syndrome and Addison's disease. However, a single blood test does not necessarily indicate optimal daily adrenal function and rhythm, which is commonly tested with a saliva test four times throughout the day.

Vitamin D

This test helps determine intestinal malabsorption and vitamin D deficiency or intoxication. It's a good idea to assess your baseline level and then retest after treatment to see how well your body is absorbing this fat-soluble vitamin.

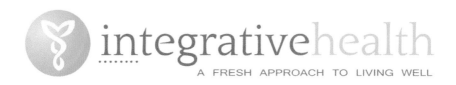

integrativehealth
A FRESH APPROACH TO LIVING WELL

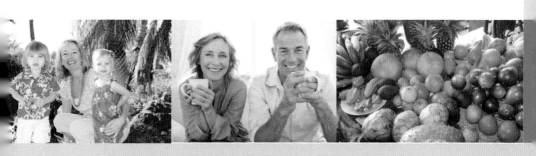

Chapter 3: Hormones

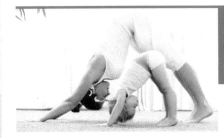

Why Hormone Balance Matters

By Dr. Adrienne Stewart

Hormones can affect our overall wellbeing. Throughout different times of our lives, hormones cycle and fluctuate. What is important is that we support the body and consider the interconnectedness and relationships of all of our hormones. All hormones in the body are designed to work together in a type of *hormonal symphony. If one member is off pitch, it affects the entire orchestra and the other members have to try to compensate.* I often describe hormone balance like sitting on a three-legged stool. The thyroid hormones are one leg of the stool, the hormones from our ovaries/testes are another, and the adrenal hormones are the third leg of the stool. It is important to assess, optimize, and balance each leg in order to sit evenly on the stool. If one leg is too long, too short or too weak, we have a lot of difficulty staying balanced and often feel like falling over!

Hormone	Deficiency Symptoms	Excess Symptoms
Thyroid	• Hair loss • Dry skin • Fatigue • Weight gain • Depression • Cold hands/feet • Constipation • Weakness	• Heart palpitations • Weight loss • Insomnia • Bone mineral loss • Thyroid eye disease • Thyroid dermopathy (pretibial myxedema) • Fatigue
Estrogen	• Vaginal dryness • Night sweats • Painful intercourse • Fatigue • Foggy thinking • Waning memory • Emotional fragility • Depression/anxiety • Achy joints • Bladder infections	• Bloating, fluid retention • Weight gain • Breast tenderness • Mood swings • Heavy bleeding/ spotting • Fibroids, endometriosis • PMS • Migraines/headaches • Breast/endometrial cancer • Gallstones • Blood clots • Nausea

Hormone	Deficiency Symptoms	Excess Symptoms
Progesterone	• PMS • Insomnia • Infertility, early miscarriage • Painful breasts, fibrocystic changes • Weight gain • Cyclic headaches • Anxiety • Hot flashes • Irregular menses or heavy menses	• Breast heaviness/ tenderness • Sleepiness, lethargy • Edema • Bloating, fullness, and constipation by slowing GI transport • Mild depression • Candida • Nausea • Spotting • Headaches • Insulin resistance • Elevated cortisol • Increased fat storage • Ligament laxity and aches • Gingivitis
Testosterone	• Persistent fatigue • Bone loss • Hot flashes • Low libido • Low motivation • Dry eyes • Vaginal dryness • Sleep disturbances • Worsening of congestive heart failure	• Acne, greasy skin/ hair • Male pattern baldness • Abnormal hair growth • Hypoglycemia • Unstable blood sugar • Thinning Hair • Infertility • Agitation/ irritability • Mid-cycle pain • Deepening voice • Clitoral enlargement • Shrinking breasts • Ovarian cysts/ PCOS
DHEA	• Adrenal dysregulation • Fatigue • Muscle weakness • Menopausal symptoms • PMS/ painful periods • Low libido • Vaginal dryness • Arthritis • Depression • Decreased appetite • Decreased memory	• Acne • Oily skin • Abnormal hair growth • Hair loss • May alter lipid profile • May increase estrogen levels • May interfere with insulin function • May potentiate the effects of PCOS • May increase mania with mood disorders

Hormone	Deficiency Symptoms	Excess Symptoms
Cortisol	• Tired and burned out • Unstable blood sugar • Foggy thinking • Low blood pressure • Thin and dry skin • Intolerance to exercise • Allergies • Difficulty fighting infection • Addison's	• Tired but wired • Sugar cravings • Lowered immunity • Cranky • Disrupted sleep • Weight gain, especially in abdomen • Skin thinning • Buffalo hump • Hypokalemia • Muscle wasting • Cushing's

All of the possible effects of hormonal dysregulation can be overwhelming and confusing. The great news is that the doctors at Integrative Health are here to help. We have many treatment options, including specific lifestyle recommendations, targeted nutrients, herbal/botanical support, and several delivery and dosage options for bioidentical hormone replacement ranging from creams, capsules, injections, to pellets. One size does not fit all in regard to hormones, so it is important to customize and personalize to each individual patient.

Hormone	Role in Body	Uses
Thyroid	• Regulates the energy level, growth, and reproduction of every cell (brain, heart, lungs, liver, skin, tissues, and all other body parts)	Improves • Metabolism • Energy • Regular bowel movements • Dry skin and dry hair • Mood
Estrogen	• 400+ functions in the body • Produced primarily by the ovaries and some produced in the liver, adrenals, breasts, and fat cells. • Proliferates endometrium • Maintains elasticity of arteries • Dilates blood vessels • Enhances blood flow • Decreases blood pressure • Stimulates endometrial growth, thickens the vaginal wall and increases uterine growth • Increases bone formation	Improves • Hot flashes • Mood swings • Memory problems • Night sweats • Vaginal dryness • Irregular menses • Painful intercourse • Low libido • Bone loss • Dry skin • Yeast infections • Headaches • Urinary tract health

Hormone	Role in Body	Uses
Progesterone	• Produced in the ovaries, the adrenal glands and, during pregnancy, in the placenta • Derived from cholesterol • Maintains uterine endometrium • Utilizes fat for energy • Natural diuretic • Helps normalize blood sugar • Lowers cholesterol • Increases core temperature during ovulation • Anti-inflammatory • Lowers blood pressure • Normalizes blood clotting and vascular tone • Reduces spasm and relaxes smooth muscle • Reduces gallbladder activity	Improves • Sleep • Estrogen dominance • Blood sugar • Swollen breasts • Headaches • Anxiety • Depression • Mood swings • Irregular menses • Cramping • Joint pain • Acne • Weight gain • Low libido • Fuzzy thinking • Bone mineral density • Cholesterol • Enhances beneficial effects of estrogen on blood vessels
Testosterone	• Secreted mainly by the testicles in males and ovaries in females and some in the adrenal glands • Sexual desire and sensation • Muscle, bone and tissue strength • Development of male reproductive tissues and sperm development • Promotes growth of body hair	Improves • Energy • Muscle weakness/ aches • Endurance • Sex drive • Bone loss • Mood • Vaginal dryness • Thinning skin • Overall wellbeing • Motivation • Memory • Heart palpitations and angina • Incontinence • Inflammation • Opposes estradiol induced breast stimulation and risks of breast cancer • Slight decrease in risk of heart attack

Hormone	Role in Body	Uses
DHEA	• Natural steroid hormone produced by the adrenal glands, gonads and the brain • Precursor of testosterone and estrogen	Improves • Energy • Lipid and insulin levels • Bone mineral density • Overall wellbeing • Other hormone levels, including testosterone and estrogens
Cortisol	• Main stress hormone • Produced by the adrenal glands • Raises blood glucose • Raises blood pressure • Mediates inflammation • Aids in metabolism • Modulates the immune system	Improves • Sleep patterns • Stress response • Energy levels • Weight control

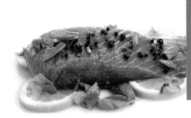

Shedding Weight with Hormonal Balance

By Dr. Alan Christianson

What's going on? You're taking all the right steps, eating healthy foods, and being consistent with your exercise routine, but the scale just won't budge. Why?

The honest-to-goodness biggest culprit? Your hormones may need some fine-tuning.

Good nutrition (proteins, healthy fats, fruits, vegetables, and whole grains) is key to helping your body make the hormones you need. If your body cannot make hormones, then it cannot be in balance. If it's not in balance, you'll be wearing your fat jeans for longer than you'd like.

So, focus on adding foods with good fats such as salmon, walnuts, and avocados to your diet. Pair these good fats with dark leafy greens such as kale, spinach, and asparagus. Snack on vitamin-rich fruits such as blueberries and bananas to give your body the nutrients it needs to stay in balance. Which hormones does your body use to stay in balance and help you achieve and maintain a healthy weight?

1. **Thyroid hormones** produce hormones that control how your body converts calories into energy. When they are too low, the calories turn straight to fat leaving you tired and heavy! Weight gain can be an indicator of an underactive thyroid gland (hypothyroidism). When the thyroid gland is underactive, your metabolism is not burning as many calories as it normally would. You also do not have as much energy, which can make it harder to get out and exercise. Other indicators of thyroid problems include dry skin, brittle nails, achy joints, and constipation. To help your thyroid, be sure to take a multivitamin with 100-200 mcg of iodine and 200 mcg of selenium. Iodized salt and brazil nuts are also great sources of these thyroid-friendly minerals.

2. **Adrenal hormones** produce cortisol, a hormone that is elevated in stressful situations. The crazy thing is that either too much or too little of this can cause weight to hang on. Some of us lead such stressful lives that our cortisol levels are always high. Eating fast food and simple carbs stress your adrenals, which increases your cortisol levels. This can lead to weight gain, especially around the midsection. Conversely, if you are not producing enough cortisol, you may have trouble getting out of bed in the morning or you may not have enough energy to make it through the day, much less exercise. When you're tired and sluggish, you tend to crave sugar and simple carbs because they give you quick energy. Ironically, the sugar and simple carbs deplete the adrenal glands making you even more tired and sluggish. Your adrenals are happy when you are! Take time for fun and rest. Try to be consistent about what time you eat your meals, sleep and wake up. Eating smaller meals every several hours can also help if your adrenals are weak.

Hormone Modification

It's difficult to obtain and maintain hormone balance without lifestyle modification. Every one of us needs to manage stress in our lives, eat a healthy diet, and exercise regularly.

3. **Reproductive hormones** are important whether you are male or female, and the right balance is important for more than your libido. Estrogen, progesterone, and testosterone are all key in keeping extra weight off.

Adrenal problems can affect the synthesis of sex hormones. The adrenals produce large amounts of DHEA, which is converted to testosterone and estrogen. Stressed adrenal glands produce too much DHEA and depleted adrenal glands don't produce enough. Weight gain may be a symptom of too much estrogen or too little progesterone in women or not enough testosterone in men. Testosterone helps maintain lean muscle mass, and low levels are also linked to lack of motivation in men. If you think these are waning, exercise is the best home remedy. Don't expect hours of plodding on the treadmill to help. Train at high intensity for shorter bursts and challenge yourself with fewer repetitions of heavier weights.

For all of these hormones, if the home measures are not doing the job, any of our docs can help out.

Listen, it's difficult to obtain and maintain hormone balance without lifestyle modification. Every one of us needs to manage stress in our lives, eat a healthy diet, and exercise regularly. Make sure that you're getting proper nutritional supplementation including adrenal and thyroid support. When your body is in balance nutritionally and hormonally, then it can balance itself physically.

Skinny jeans anyone?

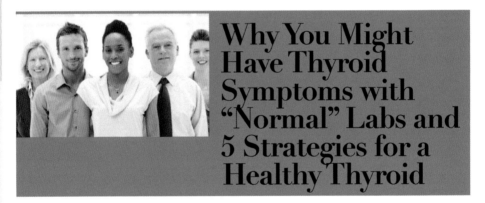

Why You Might Have Thyroid Symptoms with "Normal" Labs and 5 Strategies for a Healthy Thyroid

By Dr. Alan Christianson

For a gland that weighs about an ounce, your thyroid plays numerous fundamental roles in your body. If you have hypothyroidism, for instance, you know how frustrating fat loss can be. A sluggish thyroid can also make you tired and depressed. Do you have poor memory, dry skin, or hair loss? Your thyroid could be a major culprit.

At least 10% of adults have thyroid disease. An additional 10 – 15% have early thyroid disease, but they test within the "normal" range, and doctors don't diagnose them.

Despite showing symptoms of early thyroid disease, doctors often dismiss patients with "normal" thyroid function, and their symptoms remain. So if that person suffers from depression, a doctor might eventually prescribe Prozac rather than address thyroid deficiencies.

Why are so many people not diagnosed, and why are about 50% of those being treated for thyroid issues not feeling better?

Doctors have a normal range of numbers they use for thyroid tests. Out of 10,000 scores, they will deviate the lowest and highest 2.5 percent of these scores. But these "normal" ranges reflect the averages of all people who have had lab blood work analyzed over the last year. Many of them either had thyroid disease or potential thyroid disease.

In other words, doctors don't necessarily look at healthy people. Because many people who suffer from thyroid imbalances fall outside this pathological range, doctors don't diagnose them and so their symptoms linger.

Thyroid Imbalance

Many people who suffer from thyroid imbalances fall outside the "normal" pathological range, so doctors don't diagnose them and their symptoms linger.

Many doctors only use thyroid stimulating hormone (TSH) and T4 (your inactive form of thyroid hormone) tests. But to get a fuller picture of your thyroid issues, find a practitioner who will run a complete panel of tests including thyroid antibodies and free T3.

Testing for thyroid antibodies can rule out autoimmune diseases like Hashimoto's, a disease where your body attacks your thyroid gland. Hashimoto's is the most common cause of hypothyroidism in the U.S., yet sadly many doctors fail to diagnose this disease.

Look for your TSH to be in the optimal range of 0.3 - 1.5. If it isn't, or if other tests are abnormal, you may benefit from thyroid treatment.

Whether or not you have thyroid disease, you need to take care of this workhorse gland so it can fulfill its many duties. I want to give you five easy strategies you can use right now to improve your thyroid function:

1. **Get the right amount of iodine.** Always choose iodized salt, preferably iodized sea salt. Any salt you get in processed foods and restaurants gives you too much sodium but no iodine. On the other hand, whole foods like seafood, including wild salmon and shellfish, provide iodine. And when

you eat sushi, add some iodine-packed seaweed. I also recommend a multivitamin that contains about 100 mcg of iodine. Iodine is not a more-is-better mineral: too much, such as what you get in kelp and iodine supplements, becomes as bad or worse than too little.

2. **Get adequate selenium.** This mineral helps your body better utilize thyroid hormones. A few Brazil nuts or a good multivitamin can give you a therapeutic 200 mcg. Like iodine, selenium is not something you want too much of.

3. **Minimize mercury.** I want you to eat plenty of seafood, though unfortunately most seafood – especially larger fish, like swordfish – is packed with mercury. Many people like tuna but worry about mercury levels. I recommend eating it once a week. For the most complete current data, visit the FDA's website. I also want you to get porcelain or ceramic rather than mercury amalgams. If you have mercury amalgams (fillings), ask your dentist about removing them and then visit a specialist who focuses on mercury detoxification.

4. **Avoid perchlorate.** This toxic by-product from rocket and jet fuels ends up in your water. You also absorb it from your skin and intestines. Once in your body, perchlorate prevents your thyroid glands from absorbing iodine. To remedy this problem, I want you to drink purified rather than tap water. Ideally, use a filter for your shower also. Dry cleaning also contains perchlorate, so take your clothes out of the bag immediately and let them air out in the sunshine for a few hours before wearing.

5. **Exercise.** Step up your gym time and decrease your risk for thyroid disease. For best effect, it should be intense workouts. A study in the journal *Neuroendocrinology Letters*, for instance, found maximal aerobic exercise significantly benefits your level of circulating thyroid hormones. I love burst training and weight resistance. It's effective, efficient, and you can knock it out in just 15 minutes.

Always remember that if you suspect you might have thyroid disease or any other symptom, you never need to suffer. Educate yourself and take action. *You deserve to feel your best!*

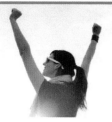

Adrenal Health

By Dr. Adrienne Stewart

Healthy adrenal glands are critical for maintaining high energy levels, resilience to stress, and hormone balance. These small organs sit on top of our kidneys and help make a large range of hormones such as DHEA, cortisol, and pregnenolone, all of which are critical for maintaining energy levels, mood balance, blood sugar levels, and proper stress response.

The adrenals help regulate our primary stress responses, giving us energy to complete tasks and even regulating immunity and reducing inflammation. Unfortunately, overstimulation of the adrenal glands over a long period of time can wear them down and cause dysfunction. Poor adrenal health is becoming more common in our modern world because of the way our bodies interpret stress. Our adrenals were designed to respond to high stress levels in short bursts because it helped our ancestors survive. Our bodies are not good at distinguishing between life and death stress and the daily emotional grind we face today. To the adrenal glands, all stress is treated the same. Chronic long-term stress that comes with modern life can create a cycle that causes the adrenals to become fatigued. When this happens, we can experience low energy, foggy thinking, muscle weakness, depression, lowered immunity, sleep disturbances, and problems regulating our blood sugar and blood pressure.

If you suspect you might have an imbalance in your adrenals, it is important to consult with your doctor at Integrative Health. We can help evaluate your adrenal health by looking at your cortisol and DHEA levels, and overall symptoms. We will create a custom health plan based on your unique picture of health that can include herbal adaptogens, nutritional support, and lifestyle changes. Because the function of the adrenals is so diverse and critical to optimal health, it is important to get evaluated. In general, though, anyone can improve their adrenal health by keeping a regular schedule of high quality sleep, eating a diet full of lean protein, fiber, and fresh vegetables, and practicing stress-reduction techniques such as yoga, meditation, or journaling.

Adrenal Hormone	Role in Body	Uses	Deficiency Symptoms	Excess Symptoms
DHEA	• Natural steroid hormone • Produced by the adrenal glands, gonads and the brain • Precursor of testosterone and estrogen	Improves • Energy • Lipid and insulin levels • Bone mineral density • Overall wellbeing • Other hormone levels including testosterone and estrogens	• Adrenal dysregulation • Fatigue • Muscle weakness • Menopausal symptoms • PMS/ painful periods • Low libido • Vaginal dryness • Arthritis • Depression • Decreased appetite • Decreased memory	• Acne • Oily skin • Abnormal hair growth • Hair loss • May alter lipid profile • May increase estrogen levels • May interfere with insulin function • May potentiate the effects of PCOS • May increase mania with mood disorders
Cortisol	• Main stress hormone • Raises blood glucose • Raises blood pressure • Mediates inflammation • Aids in metabolism • Modulates the immune system	Improves • Sleep patterns • Stress response • Energy levels • Weight control	• Tired and burned out • Unstable blood sugar • Foggy thinking • Low blood pressure • Thin and dry skin • Intolerance to exercise • Allergies • Difficulty fighting infection • Addison's	• Tired but wired • Sugar cravings • Lowered immunity • Cranky • Disrupted sleep • Weight gain, especially in abdomen • Skin thinning • Buffalo hump • Hypokalemia • Muscle wasting • Cushing's

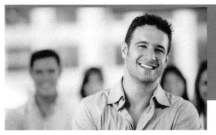

Man Up When it Comes to Your Health

By Dr. Linda Khoshaba

The hottest trend in men's wellness is focused on a condition known as hypogonadism. Hypogonadism is a condition in which the testes or pituitary gland do not make enough male sex hormones, especially testosterone. While most men do not want to hear that peak testosterone occurs around 18 years of age, it's true! Testosterone levels then begin to plateau in the twenties and then begin to decline by 1.5% each year, starting at 30 years of age. By the time a man is in his eighties, he will have half the amount of testosterone he had when he was 18.

What are signs and symptoms of Hypogonadism?
Signs of male hypogonadism include fatigue, depression, irritability, difficulty concentrating, poor exercise recovery, poor muscle mass, erectile dysfunction and impaired libido. This condition can be treated and has a good prognosis.

Explaining Male Hormone Levels and Ranges
It's not a bad idea to get your male hormone levels measured to see if you are at risk for hypogonadism. Ask your doctor to run a male hormone panel to determine your current blood levels. Male hormones include free and total Testosterone, DHEA, Dihydrotestosterone (DHT), and Androstenedione. In addition, Prostate Specific Antigen (PSA) should also be a part of the lab workup for hypogonadism.

Free vs. Total vs. Bioavailable Testosterone
There are two main ways to test blood levels of testosterone: free and total. Free testosterone means that the hormone is not bound to albumin, a blood plasma protein, and makes up the small percentage (1-4%) of what is available to use. Total testosterone is bound to albumin and another protein known as Sex Hormone Binding Globulin (SHBG) and makes up about 98% of testosterone in your body. Since total testosterone is loosely bound to albumin, it can easily be unbound and, together with free testosterone, becomes bioavailable testosterone.

Optimal versus standard broad reference ranges are outlined below.
- Optimal Total testosterone levels are between 790-1100ng/dL (280-800ng/dL is a standard reference range)
- Optimal Free testosterone levels are between 20-35 pg/dL (8-30 pg/dL is a standard reference range)

- Optimal Bioavailable testosterone levels are between 400-640pg/dL (120-600pg/dL is a standard reference range)

Treatment Options

There are many different types of testosterone treatments available for hypogonadism. There are oral, sublingual, topical, injections, and subdermal ways to administer testosterone replacement therapy.

Testosterone Treatments

There are many different types of testosterone treatments available for hypogonadism. There are oral, sublingual, topical, injections, and subdermal ways to administer testosterone replacement therapy.

Although most of these delivery methods can help, the most effective way to stabilize testosterone levels in the blood, which has the best compliance rate, is subdermal, also known as pellet therapy. Unlike oral testosterone that has to be broken down by the liver first, pellet therapy is great because it bypasses the liver, does not affect clotting factors, and does not increase risk of thrombosis. Overall, pellet therapy has a better efficacy rate and has a lower side effect profile.

Doesn't testosterone therapy cause Prostate Cancer?

This is the main question that comes up when discussing testosterone replacement therapy. According to several longitudinal studies, testosterone causing prostate cancer is a myth. The notion that testosterone increases prostate cancer stems from one journal article that showed giving testosterone to one patient with existing metastatic prostate cancer worsened his prognosis. Recent data from numerous clinical trials have shown no increases in rates of prostate cancer with testosterone supplementation in normal men and in men with increased risk for prostate cancer.

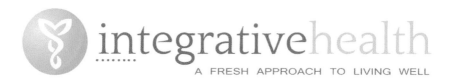

integrativehealth
A FRESH APPROACH TO LIVING WELL

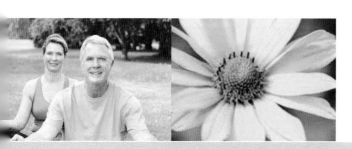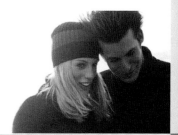

Chapter 4: Seasonal

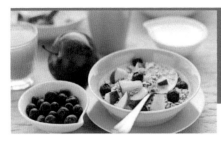

Reshaping for the New Year: Part One

By Dr. Saman Rezaie

It's a new year, the resolutions abound and weight loss is on top of the list. We will be covering how to jump-start the goal for losing weight in two parts. The first part is going to cover tips for getting your diet into shape, and the second part will cover exercise.

You want to make changes to your body and lose weight, so the real change begins with your diet. We are going to take a look at some areas you can tweak that will bring about the biggest changes for you.

Breakfast

This is the most important meal of the day for a reason. You constantly see research about how some foods are good for you, then bad, and then back to good again. However, there has never been anything that says breakfast is bad. Breakfast sets the tone for your whole day. The most common mistake is skipping your first meal of the day. You need to have breakfast within one hour of waking up to start your metabolism. You want your breakfast to pack 20 grams of protein and a portion of slow-releasing carbohydrates to balance blood sugars through the morning and send your body into weight loss mode. All this makes a big difference for your blood sugars, cortisol levels, stress management, metabolism, and energy throughout the day. Starting your day off with the right meal can elevate your whole day and strengthen your body.

Nutrient-Dense Foods

What are nutrient-dense foods? There are two big areas of this category, macronutrients and micronutrients. Macronutrients are proteins, fats, and carbohydrates. These are important for our body because they are the fuel for our metabolism. Micronutrients are the vitamins and minerals that act as co-factors to help metabolize the macronutrients. The current diet trends have people eating a macronutrient-dense diet, which is great because you are getting large amounts of energy and creating satiety. The problem with these macronutrient-dense diets is that your body is micronutrient starved, causing your body to still be hungry and store more fat. Implement this second dietary habit of consuming nutrient-dense foods to nourish your body and shed pounds. Ever hear, "taste the rainbow?" Forget the Skittles® and apply the phrase to all the differently colored foods Mother Nature has to offer, and your body will thank you.

Calorie Count

What is a calorie and why is everyone so concerned about them? Ever hear about calories in and calories out? Well, this is not the standard anymore. The problem is that people are eating foods that have so many calories packed into them, that they are eating less food, but getting more calories into their bodies. If the calories you were ingesting were packed with vitamins and minerals, you would not have to eat as much food to be full. Your body would also be more efficient at processing the fuel it was given, because it has all of the tools that it needs to process and produce the largest output of energy from the least amount of food. So, the lesson here is that quality over quantity is the key. As you implement quality food into your diet, you will find that the amount of food does not matter as much and, more importantly, you won't need such calorie dense foods.

Clean it up

Clean up your diet and get the gunk out of your system for your body to function at an optimal level and burn fat. To clear your system for a fresh start, you must remove all the sugars, alcohol, preservatives, artificial sweeteners, etc. All of these are harming your body, without you even realizing it. They are causing inflammation throughout the body, hormone dysregulation, and throwing off your gut bacteria. Do you ever feel bloated, tired, or your bowels just aren't working right? By removing all the aforementioned items, you will decrease the inflammation happening in your GI tract and immune system that is causing you to carry excess body weight and making you more susceptible to diseases. Cleaning up your diet will also harmonize your hormones, giving you optimal energy levels, and balance out the bacteria in your gut. Researchers are now finding that certain bacteria in the digestive tracts are involved in keeping us obese and others are involved in keeping us thin, so it's very important to have a healthy flora balance.

Clean It Up

Clean up your diet and get the gunk out of your system for your body to function at an optimal level and burn fat. To clear your system for a fresh start, you must remove all of the sugars, alcohol, preservatives, artificial sweeteners, etc.

This has been Part One of Reshaping for the New Year for a new you. Stay tuned for Part Two, where we will discuss which exercises will help you get back into your skinny jeans.

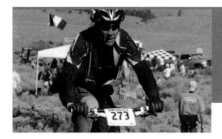

Reshaping for the New Year: Part Two

By Dr. Saman Rezaie

It is a new year, the resolutions abound and weight loss is on the top of the list. We started with Part One and covered diet because it has the most immediate impact on your health, yielding changes for you to see in a few days. Recent research has shown that exercise is just as important as a healthy diet, so in Part Two we will cover how to jump-start weight loss with exercise. Now that you have some dietary changes in place and have started to see some pounds drop off, it is time to get started on your workout routine. Building more muscle will increase your metabolism and help burn off that adipose tissue. Here are the best tips that you can put into place to lose weight, and get healthy and happy.

Start Slowly

This is the biggest key to getting into a workout routine, and actually staying in your workout routine. I know you are super excited about getting back into working out, and maybe, at some point, you even used to work out every day. Remember, you have taken some time off from exercising, so take some time to get back into it every day. You can achieve effective weight loss with 30 minutes of exercise, three times per week. Start out with mild to moderate exercise a few times per week, allowing your body to recover with a day of rest. Giving your body recovery time is important to avoid injury, because too much, too soon can put you on the sidelines and not on the weight loss team. Injuries come from misuse and overuse, so start out smart and give your body a chance. Once you are able to do three times per week with no major problem, start to increase the number of days you work out per week, or start increasing your intensity of exercise.

Intensity

Are you doing cardio for 30 minutes? One hour? More than one hour? Still not seeing the results that you want from your exercise? Here's a tip: the intensity of your workout is one of the biggest factors for achieving weight loss. Duration is not as important. So, the people who work out out the hardest, not the longest, are allowing for the best weight loss. Workouts are starting to go toward high intensity interval training (HIIT), Peak 8, Orangetheory, and burst training, with more to come. The goal is to produce intervals of your highest intensity with a lower intensity period between them. This allows for an increased demand on your heart, muscles, and metabolism. This is a must-add to your workout but, as we mentioned above, start out slowly and build up the amount of time you are doing the intensity and intervals.

Muscle Confusion

Another aspect of your new workout that will benefit you for weight loss is muscle confusion, like P90X, CrossFit, and other workout forms. This is based on doing a variety of exercises to stress your muscles in new ways, allowing for more growth, which will also stimulate your metabolism to allow for more weight loss. If you are walking all the time, adding in a day of bike riding, hiking, or even yoga can be a simple way to cross train. This allows some muscle confusion so your body does not get used to the same thing over and over, producing fewer results over time than when you first started the routine. When you start with a new exercise, start slowly and increase the intensity as you get the hang of it.

Get out there with the second phase of your weight loss program. The combination of diet and exercise has the most dramatic impact on your mind, body and achieving the weight loss goals you desire. So, start out slowly, add the intensity, and eventually some variety, to produce the best results!

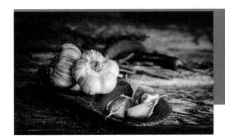

Fight Colds & Flu with Fresh Veggies

By Dr. Linda Khoshaba

When we are officially in the flu season, it is important that you keep your immune system healthy so you can fight off any bug that you may encounter. Here are the top 5 foods that will boost your immune system and help you survive this winter season. The best part is that you can make a dish that combines all 5 of these foods and use it as anti-flu and anti-cold remedy!

1. Garlic (Latin Name: Allium Sativa)

Garlic comes from the Liliaceae family and is usually used in its bulb form. Garlic is known for its powerful taste and smell, which is mainly due to sulfur-containing compounds known as allicin.

Garlic has numerous immune-stimulating properties, including being a powerful diaphoretic, which makes you sweat, and an antimicrobial agent. It can also be combined with other compounds, such as mullein oil, and be used as ear drops to treat ear infections. As a food, its pungent taste will go great in any soup and will definitely increase circulation. If you are brave enough, try eating one clove per day for preventative purposes, but make sure you have some mouthwash nearby.

2. Onions (Latin Name: Allium Cepa)
Onions come from the same family as Garlic and also contain sulfur-containing compounds. They contain a little less sulfur, although it may not seem that way because cutting raw onions can sometimes make you cry. Traditionally, onions have been used in many contexts, including mild infections, coughs, and colds, because of their antibacterial actions. Recently, research has shown that onions contain some of the richest sources of dietary flavonoids, one of the most abundant being Quercetin. These flavonoids have great antioxidant and anti-inflammatory effects and work by inhibiting the release of mediators of inflammation such as histamine from white blood cells. Onions are also very powerful in helping to reduce allergies and asthma.

3. Turmeric (Botanical Name: Curcuma Longa)
This root has been historically linked to countries such as India and China, and has been well known for anti-inflammatory effects on autoimmune conditions such as rheumatoid arthritis. The active constituent, curcumin, makes turmeric such a top a candidate across the board for numerous health conditions. Turmeric resembles ginger root because they both come from the same Zingiberaceae family. It has a distinctive yellow-orange color and, because the pigment is so bright, it has historically been used as a dye for clothing. Turmeric possesses many antiviral properties and can help fight off influenza.

4. Ginger (Botanical Name: Zingiber)
Ginger has many beneficial uses. There are numerous clinical research findings to show ginger's efficacy in treatment and prophylaxis for motion sickness and nausea. Ginger is very warming and can be great for warming up cold extremities. Ginger tastes wonderful in foods such as stir-fry and soups.

5. Lemon (Botanical Name: Citrus x limon)
Lemon with honey is a very common remedy used for cold and flu. Lemon comes from the Citrus family and has a reputation for containing excellent sources of Vitamin C. Vitamin C itself has many notable immune modulating effects, working as a natural antihistamine and helping to keep the immune cells in check. This vitamin has many soothing properties to help treat a sore throat and calm congestion.

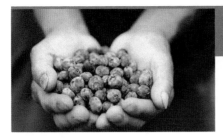

Spring Detox

By Dr. Alan Christianson

Health savvy people know that Spring cleaning is about more than your garage. Every day we are all exposed to thousands of factors that disrupt our health. Since 1900, chemists have created over 3 million new chemicals that our bodies may not be adapted to. Some are really dangerous because we cannot get rid of them very well. This means that even if we are exposed to only tiny amounts, they can build up over time, just like a thick layer of dust in a vacant home. Some of the worst chemicals that do this include metals like mercury, pesticides like 2, 4-D, and plastic byproducts like BPA.

Chemicals like these are thought to be factors behind most chronic diseases, including:	Along with devastating long-term effects, these chemicals can also factor into daily health concerns, such as:
Diabetes Many cancers Heart disease Alzheimer's disease	Obesity Fatigue Depression Arthritis Muscular pain Short-term memory losses

Springtime is always a great time to turn over a new leaf and amp up your health to a whole new level. Here are my **10 favorite tricks to detox** right this year:

Pre-tox is the theme for the first steps. To get toxins out of your body, you first want to reduce the number of toxins coming in.

1. Learn when organic matters
Some foods, like celery, blueberries, butter, and coffee are critical to get in organic versions. Other foods, like sweet potatoes, oranges or white meat poultry are less critical.

2. Don't pollute yourself by cleaning your home
Avoid strong smelling cleaners. Nearly everything can be cleaned with simple things like Castile soap, vinegar, and citrus extracts.

3. Take a breath of fresh air

The largest source of toxins for all of us is the air we breathe in our homes. Use HEPA air filters or ionizers and have your ducts cleaned each year. Re-tox is one of the biggest problems of chemical exposure. Our detox systems are just not set up to deal with the type of toxins we are exposed to. As we try to get the toxins out, we can make them more dangerous and send them into our vital tissues like our brain and thyroid. This has been called the problem of Re-Tox. How can you stop it?

4. H2O

How much do you need? Most of us should drink at least half our body weight in ounces each day.

5. RBF

All the toxins trying to get out are coming back in through your colon. Rice bran fiber can help. Add 1 tablespoon per day to your breakfast shake.

6. Chlorophyll

The greener your poop is, the cleaner your body will be. Chlorophyll is the green pigment in plant foods. No, green Skittles® do not count. To get green, eat at least 3 cups per day of kale, spinach, or collards.

Active Detox. The next three steps are for a targeted detox process done over a period of two weeks. This can reduce your chemical burden and help you thrive in no time.

Detox Shake

For advanced detox and weight loss, have this for lunch also!

7. Detox shake

For breakfast, make up a mix of:

1 serving unsweetened vegetable based protein powder

1 Tbs. chia seeds

1 Tbs. rice bran fiber

1 cup berries

½ cup frozen spinach

1 cup unsweetened coconut beverage

For advanced detox and weight loss, have this for lunch also.

8. Rest your insides

During the cleanse, have 1-2 lean and green meals with your shake. These would be lean protein plus steamed vegetables or salad vegetables. Avoid all other food during the cleanse.

9. Detoxing light pollution

You detox better when your circadian rhythms are in sync. During the cleanse, make your mornings bright. This means that within one hour of waking up, expose yourself to sunlight for 30 minutes. Even if it is cold and cloudy, the sunlight is thousands of times more powerful than the brightest indoor light.

10. Social detox

The best way to stay healthy is to hang out with healthy people. Make new health-conscious friends, and teach your old friends your new tricks!

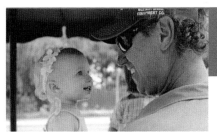

Summer Living

By Dr. Linda Khoshaba

Summer is finally here; time for some fun in the sun! Here are three summer tips to help you prepare and have a successful and safe summer.

1. Summer Sweats

With the temperature rising, making sure you get adequate hydration is probably the top priority for keeping your body fluids in balance. Appropriate water intake consists of drinking at least half your body weight in ounces, and more for every hour of physical activity. When you perspire, the content mostly consists of water and, to lesser extent, minerals such as sodium, potassium, calcium and magnesium. It is essential that not only is water replaced, but also to make sure your electrolyte replacement is sufficient. Electrolytes are responsible for balancing pH levels (blood acidity) and regulating muscle function. Common electrolyte replacements are drinks such as Gatorade, however, be cautious with the sugar content hidden in these drinks. Instead, consider adding drinks such as Emergen-C® or Endurolytes® Fizz that do not contain refined sugars and additives.

2. Simple Summer Sweets

Ice pops can be refreshing, but be cautious of sugar content! You can make ice treats without overindulging in calories. Cut up some pieces of fruit such as peaches, kiwi, strawberries, and grapes, add some water, fill up a popsicle tray, and then freeze. Another thirst quencher is to make some old-fashioned lemonade. All you need to do is cut 5 lemons in half, squeeze them, and then add the juice to a pitcher of water and ice! Not only will this keep you hydrated, it is amazingly low in calories!

3. Summer Skin Care

Skin is our body's largest organ. Before jumping into your swimsuit, think about how you can protect your skin! Sun protection factor (SPF) is a rating that measures the amount of time it takes to form a sunburn on unprotected skin. However, this factor only measures UVB rays (short rays), not UVA rays (long rays). UVA rays penetrate deeper layers of skin and UVB rays penetrate the skin more superficially. It is important to protect yourself from both forms of ultraviolet radiation, as they both can increase your risk of premature aging, wrinkles, and skin cancers. Here is what can you do to protect yourself from sun damage:

Try to hang out in the shade, especially between the hours of 10 am and 4 pm.

Choosing your outdoor clothing wisely can reduce your risk as well. For example, there are clothes that designed to reflect UV light, reducing skin exposure.

The color of your clothes can impact how much radiation you are absorbing; brighter and dark-colored clothes reflect more UV than light pastel colored clothes.

Avoid tanning booths.

Look for a sunscreen with SPF over 15 and with protection from both UVA and UVB rays.

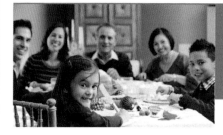

Thriving Under Holiday Stress

By Dr. Linda Khoshaba

'Tis the season that you're overloaded with great food, company, and stress! It may seem impossible to overcome because you're easily sidetracked from your regular eating and exercising routines; however, it can be simple to maintain your health with some quick and easy suggestions.

Exercise BEFORE Dining

If you know that a holiday dinner party is coming up, plan a workout **before** the dinner. Try to spend at least 30-45 minutes engaged in aerobic and anaerobic high intensity interval training (HIIT) exercises. Aerobic exercises include running, walking, dancing, swimming, hiking, biking, or using the treadmill and elliptical machines, to name a few. Anaerobic exercises include sprinting and weight lifting. Together, these exercise strategies increase your heart rate, speeding up the burning of fat and glucose. Your delicious holiday meal will replenish the calories and energy burned through exercise.

Savor the Meal

As you sit down to enjoy this holiday meal, remember to slow down and take pleasure in the experience instead of finishing like it's a food marathon. Not only does slowing down improve digestion by helping you chew your food longer, it has also been shown to help you shed pounds! This mastication method will prevent overeating and help your brain process two important hormones involved in eating, Ghrelin and Leptin. Ghrelin signals the stomach to continue sending hunger messages to the brain, while Leptin signals the brain that satiety is reached. In the long run, you will eat less, and both your stomach and body will thank you for it later.

Remember to Breathe

The hectic season is upon us, causing stress levels to rise. Stress can be caused by time constraints, changes in your routine, and the rush to meet deadlines. A 2 to 5 minute daily deep breathing exercise can help you cope with these times. Even a 15-minute "de-stress" session by yourself with no distractions can reset your mind so you can handle the stress. Stress will always be there; it is how you deal with it that makes a difference in your health. There are great ways to incorporate rest and relaxation into your holiday season, like reading, yoga, meditation, and breathing exercises. With the abundance of technology today, there are even applications you can download to help you relax.

Savor the Meal

As you sit down to enjoy this holiday meal, remember to slow down and take pleasure in the experience instead of finishing like it's a food marathon.

Don't Sacrifice Sleep

Sleep is essential to your daily functioning, but during the holidays it is too easy to sacrifice this critical process. With lots of family and friends around, you steer away from regular bedtime schedules. Getting at least 7 to 8 hours of quality sleep will help you function better, improve your metabolism, and help you keep the weight off. Even taking a short nap during the day can invigorate and refresh your mind. With proper rest, you will be more productive throughout the day and have more time to spend with loved ones. Keep in mind that it is the quality of sleep that counts, not the quantity. To improve your quality of sleep, avoid caffeinated products, alcohol, and eating late in the evening. A nice Epsom salt bath at least 30 minutes before bed promotes a relaxing sleep thanks to the magnesium content that acts as a muscle relaxant.

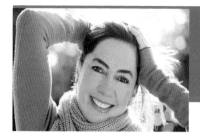

Cooling Down Holiday Hot Flashes

By Dr. Adrienne Stewart

During the holiday season, we are surrounded by the comfort and cheer of our family traditions. What many women might not know is that these very traditions could be triggering an increase in hot flashes.

Below are three common culprits for hot flashes and how to avoid them this holiday season.

Sweating Over Sweets
Sweet treats like holiday cookies, candy canes, and gingerbread houses may be holiday treats, but they can also spike your blood sugar. This dramatic fluctuation in blood sugar can affect hormone levels, which trigger the tell-tale heat of a hot flash.

To combat this common culprit, try swapping sugary sweets with healthy alternatives. If you do feel the need to indulge, try saving the sweets as a treat after a meal filled with lean protein and fiber. This will slow the absorption of the sugar, keeping your blood glucose from spiking. In a pinch, try combining the sweet with a protein such as lean turkey or some nut butter.

The Flush of Wine
Holiday toasts are a wonderful tradition; however, be careful of consuming too much alcohol. The sugars in wine and other alcoholic beverages can spike your blood sugar the same as eating a holiday cookie. In addition, the alcohol puts an extra strain on your liver that in turn affects the way your hormones are processed. Party punch spiked with alcohol is especially dangerous for triggering a hot flash.

To combat this common culprit, try limiting alcohol to a few sips. Try drinking it with a meal rich with fiber, essential fatty acids, and lean proteins to keep blood sugar stable. The best alternative is to reach for water. This will help hydrate you during the dry winter months and keep your skin glowing. A glass of green tea is another great option because it has L-Theanine, which can be relaxing and balance out the caffeine. If you're still missing the wine, try sipping on pomegranate, tart cherry, or 100% cranberry juice in a nice holiday wine glass.

The Strain of Stress

Although the holidays are about family and memories, it can also be an incredibly stressful time. From baking to shopping to extra obligations, it is no wonder our stress levels rise this time of year. Unfortunately, too much stress affects almost every system of the body in a negative way. Hormone levels can become unbalanced as our adrenal glands work overtime trying to compensate. Plus, the extra cortisol released from the adrenal glands can lead to weight gain directly around the abdomen.

To combat this common culprit, try implementing some coping strategies for holiday stress. Make sure not to overcommit or agree to too many extra obligations. Even though coffee and all the holiday caffeinated drinks may give you a short-term boost, it can trigger hot flashes and affect restorative sleep. Support your body with extra sleep and exercise. Mindful practices such as meditation and yoga can also help. And remember, you don't have to do everything. It's okay to say no, or to ask for help.

The Strain of Stress

Unfortunately, too much stress affects almost everybody's system in a negative way. Hormone levels can become unbalanced as our adrenal glands work overtime trying to compensate. Plus, the extra cortisol released from the adrenal glands can lead to weight gain directly around the abdomen.

When in Doubt, Ask for Help

If hot flashes become too troublesome, be sure to ask your naturopathic doctor about other alternatives. All of the possible effects of hormonal dysregulation can be overwhelming and confusing. The great news is that we are here to help. As naturopathic doctors, we have many treatment options that include trigger avoidance, specific lifestyle recommendations, targeted nutrients, herbal/botanical support, and delivery and dosage options for bioidentical hormone replacement. One size does not fit all in regard to hormones, so it is important to customize and personalize to your individual needs.

Healthy Holiday Muffins

This holiday muffin is a great way to start the day. The fiber from the applesauce and whole grains, essential fatty acids from the nuts and flax seeds, and cinnamon content help to keep your blood sugar and hormone levels balanced without sacrificing flavor and fun.

Healthy Holiday Muffins

This holiday muffin is a great way to start the day. The fiber from the applesauce and whole grains, essential fatty acids from the nuts and flax seeds, and cinnamon content help to keep your blood sugar and hormone levels balanced without sacrificing flavor and fun.

Ingredients:

1/4 cup organic oil (canola, sunflower seed)

1 1/4 cups organic applesauce

1 1/2 cups whole wheat pastry flour, or gluten-free pastry flour

2 Tbs. fresh ground flax seed

1/2 tsp. baking soda

1 tsp. non-aluminum baking powder

1 tsp. cinnamon

1 pinch salt

1/2 cup chopped walnuts

Directions:

Preheat oven to 375 F. Lightly coat a 12-cup muffin tin with cooking spray or paper liners.

Combine oil and applesauce. In a separate bowl, sift together the flour, ground flax, baking soda and powders, cinnamon, salt and walnuts. Stir wet and dry ingredients together until just combined. Use a large spoon to drop the muffin batter into the muffin tins. Bake 18 to 20 minutes and enjoy!

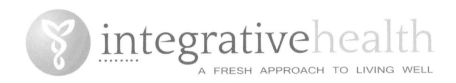

integrativehealth
A FRESH APPROACH TO LIVING WELL

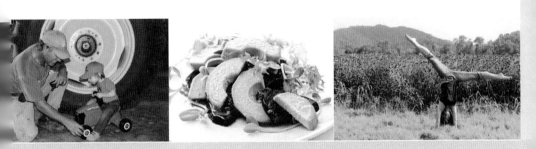

Chapter 5: Food & Nutrition

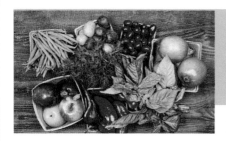

Optimal Food Guidelines

By Dr. Alan Christianson

WATER

Water is our body's principal chemical component, making up more than 60 percent of our body weight. Every system in our body depends on water. For example, water flushes toxins out of vital organs, carries nutrients to our cells, and provides a moist environment for ear, nose and throat tissues. Lack of water can lead to dehydration, and even mild dehydration can limit your bodily functions and drain your energy. Most of us get far too little water. In general, men should consume 3 liters a day (13 cups) and women 2.2 liters a day (9 cups). Requirements vary for children. Exercise, hot, humid or cold climates, illnesses or health conditions, and being pregnant or nursing all require us to increase our water intake and possibly add electrolytes to our diets. Other beverages do not count as water. Drinks with sugar or caffeine can make you lose more fluid than they provide.

HEALTH PROMOTING FOODS

Getting the bulk of your diet from the following foods is the simplest way to lower your risk of heart disease, diabetes, stroke and cancers. Your choices in diet and lifestyle are the main determinants to your health.

VEGETABLES

These are most commonly deficient in the average American diet and the most needed in our fast-paced, chemical-laced lives.

Ways to get veggies in your diet include:

Salads: Especially mixed greens, romaine or red lettuce. Avoid Iceberg.

Fresh vegetable juices: Limit if concerned about weight or blood sugar.

Soups: Frozen, packaged or make it homemade! It's easy! Just take your favorite veggies and boil them with spring water, 1 tablespoon of olive oil, and a naturally seasoned salt, like Spike®. You can make a large batch ahead of time. It will keep for up to 1 week, or you can freeze some in single serving sizes for future meals.

General Recommendations for Veggies:
Try to get 5 servings a day ~ Use many different colors in your diet ~ Experiment with specialty produce for variety, and if you see something you do not recognize, try it! ~ Organic is preferable ~ Fresh is better than frozen ~ Avoid canned

Note: Some vegetables are prone to cause high levels of insulin secretion. Eat these less often if you are concerned about your weight or if your blood sugar is unstable. Examples are beets, carrots, corn, potatoes, and squash.

FRUITS
Like vegetables, fruits are high in fiber, vitamins, and many beneficial phytochemicals.

General Recommendations for Fruit:
0-3 servings daily ~ Try to buy organic, especially for berries, grapes and dried fruits ~ Avoid exceeding 6 ounces of juice daily ~ Choose fresh over frozen, frozen over canned ~ Avoid any types with sugars or preservatives added

Fruits

Like vegetables, fruits are high in fiber, vitamins, and many beneficial phytochemicals.

Great Examples of Fruit:

Berries: All kinds are great! Strawberries, blackberries, blueberries, raspberries...

Tree fruits: Apples, avocados, apricots, nectarines, peaches, bananas, pears, blood oranges, grapefruit, lemons, limes, oranges...

Note: Fruits highest in sugar are bananas, grapes, mango, papaya, apricots, dates, prunes, raisins and other dried fruits. With dried, always choose organic and avoid those with sulfites. If your weight is too high, your blood sugar unstable, or you have intestinal infections present, you should avoid the high sugar fruit and juice, and possibly this food group altogether, until your body is in balance.

PROTEINS
Protein is such an important part of our bodies that it pays to take it seriously. We need the right amount and the correct kinds of protein to function at our best. A 180-pound man needs 65-70 grams of protein and a 135-pound woman needs about 50 grams each and every day. An ounce of lean meat, chicken, or fish has about 7 grams, a cup of either nonfat milk or soy milk has 8 grams, an egg has 6 grams, and an ounce of cheese has 6-7 grams.

General Recommendations for Proteins:
Include with all meals ~ Always choose free range and organic sources

Great Examples of Protein:
Red Meats: Buffalo, beef, lamb, rabbit, venison.

Poultry: Chicken, Cornish hens, ostrich, turkey.

Fish: Cod, herring, halibut, salmon, sardines, mahi, tuna... Include 1-3 servings per week in your diet, unless you are pregnant or nursing, then limit it to one serving per week. Even a few servings weekly can lower risks of heart disease by 50%, but do not exceed this amount significantly due to the mercury pollution of our planet. It is best to avoid freshwater fish due to mercury and pollutants.

Eggs: 0-5 per week (common food allergen)

Dairy: Cottage cheese, unsweetened yogurt, milk, cheese, yogurt (common food allergens) Rice, goat or sheep products are best.

Soy Products: Fermented types like miso, tempeh and natto are safer, but do not rely on as a sole source of protein and avoid all if pregnant or nursing.

Note: Avoid all processed meats. Choose organic and hormone free items. If you experience poor sleep or food cravings at night, avoid proteins during the evening meal and after.

Carbohydrates

Carbohydrates are large contributors of calories to a diet. Along with fat, carbs are the main source of fuel for our body.

CARBOHYDRATES
Carbohydrates are large contributors of calories to a diet. Along with fat, carbs are the main source of fuel for our body. Although intake of vegetables, proteins, and essential fats should not be reduced, carbohydrate intake can be reduced when body fat is elevated. Do not restrict intake of carbohydrates to less than 1 cup (cooked) daily.

General Recommendations for Carbs:
Whole Grain: Amaranth, brown rice, brown rice pasta, buckwheat, oatmeal, quinoa, whole rye, wild rice, and unprocessed wheat foods like wheat berries, bulgur, and whole-wheat pasta.

READ LABELS! Avoid all processed or refined grains! Watch for them in baked goods, sauces, thickeners, pastas, rice, breads, couscous and packaged foods. These foods have lost much of their nutrient value, but have retained all of their calories.

Note: Through repeated hybridization, wheat and corn have been altered more than any other foods! Wheat contains a complex protein called gliadin that worsens the health of many people. Those who are sensitive can experience symptoms as clear as life-threatening bleeding (celiac disease), or as vague as depression or fatigue (wheat allergy). Wheat is one of our most highly chemically treated food products. Symptoms from wheat may be reactions to many chemicals, like formaldehyde, used in its processing. If your health is not optimal, we encourage you to avoid wheat-containing foods for a trial period of three weeks. Testing can also be done to pinpoint those most sensitive.

Beans/Legumes: Peas, alfalfa, clover, beans, lentils, lupins, carob and peanuts. These are great sources of fiber and some vitamins, but need other nutrients to be ingested at the same time to become a complete protein.

BENEFICIAL FATS

Essential fats are one of the more common deficiencies in the American diet. Harmful fats are one of the most dangerous excesses. It is best to get your fats naturally from the foods you eat rather than adding fats to foods. When you need to add fats for cooking or on a salad, always choose good fats. And remember, a serving of fat is very small.

Beneficial Fats

Essential fats are one of the more common deficiencies in the American diet.

Good Fats to use Liberally: (2-5 servings daily) Almond oil, avocado, extra virgin olive or brown rice oils, raw seeds like flax, pumpkin, sesame and sunflower.

Good Fats to use Sparingly: (2-5 servings weekly) Eggs (free range organic), fatty fish, flaxseed oil (not for cooking), nuts (organic, raw and unsalted), organic Ghee (clarified butter), organic butter.

Note: A good Omega-3 supplement is also recommended for almost everyone. Watch what brand you use! Many contain high levels of mercury.

HEALTHFUL FLAVORINGS

Arrowroot as a thickener ~ Culinary herbs and spices ~ Himalayan salt (in moderation) ~ Stevia as a sweetener

FOODS TO AVOID

Dairy: Although much conflicting research does exist, we generally recommend against daily use of cow dairy foods. Recent studies suggest they may not even protect against osteoporosis. Dairy is a common cause of gas, bloating, nausea, nasal mucus, sinus allergies and frequent ear infections. If none of these symptoms are noticed after eating dairy foods, occasional use is all right, but use organic and hormone-free sources.

All Carbs with Gluten

Sugars and Artificial Sweeteners: Avoid or severely limit all but those naturally found in foods. These are poisons to our bodies! Check for these in all sauces, beverages, desserts, cereals, baked goods, yogurt, preserves, cakes, cookies, candies and ice cream. Look for the words high fructose corn syrup, dextrose, corn sweetener, sucrose, fructose, sucralose or Splenda®, aspartame or NutraSweet®, and anything a non-chemist can't easily pronounce.

Anything Artificial: Dyes or coloring, flavors, MSG (hidden on labels as natural flavoring or vegetable protein), preservatives, processed items like bacon, ham, lunchmeats or sausage.

Fats: Trans Fatty Acids, margarine, vegetable shortening, hydrogenated oils, fried foods, homogenized dairy.

Caffeine: One serving a day will be tolerable for most people, but more than that is generally harmful.

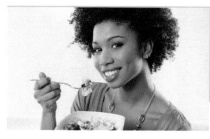

Healthy Diet Tips

By Dr. Alan Christianson

It's critical to stay on track with food decisions. Here are the most important things to keep in mind:

COMMON FOOD MYTHS

- Good food takes too much time
- Good food is more expensive
- Junk food is tastier

Thankfully, not a single one of these myths are true.

Once you learn these quick tips, you'll be eating better and spending less time in the kitchen.

Good food does not have to cost more, especially not if you factor in the savings on corrective health treatments.

Your taste buds will change in just a few weeks. If you eat clean for awhile, you really will not find processed foods appealing.

ELEMENTS OF A HEALTHY MEAL
- Produce - fresh fruits and vegetables should be about 1/2 of each meal
- Protein - should come from a variety of sources and ideally be about 1/4 of the meal
- High fiber starch - the remaining 1/4 of the meal

If there is one thing a healthy diet is not lacking, it's options.

For each of the elements mentioned above, I have compiled a list of the key concepts, along with numerous examples.

Produce - Best sources
Eat the Rainbow! Some of the most powerful nutrients in plants are the chemicals that make their colors. To get a good variety of them, try to eat something from each color group daily. What could be simpler?

Beets	Artichokes	Bananas
Cherries	Arugula	Cauliflower
Pomegranates	Broccoli	Ginger
Raspberries	Brussels Sprouts	Jicama
Red Bell Peppers	Celery	Kohlrabi
Strawberries	Cabbage	Mushrooms
Tomatoes	Leeks	Onions
	Spinach	Parsnips
	Zucchini	Turnips
Apricots	Black Currants	
Butternut Squash	Blackberries	
Carrots	Blueberries	
Lemon	Plums	
Oranges	Eggplant	
Peaches	Grapes	
Pumpkin	Purple Tomatoes	
Tangerines		
Yellow Peppers		

Produce - General Concepts	Quick Produce - Examples
Fresh or frozen Variety Rainbow Organic when possible Raw or lightly cooked	Carrot sticks Celery sticks Prepared lettuce Broccoli florets Apples Berries

After produce, the most important element in the diet is protein.

We all say we want to lose weight, but we are really trying to lose fat. Nothing helps this more than protein. Ideally, good quality protein would make up 1/4 - 1/2 of our diet.

Protein - Best Sources	Protein - Concepts	Quick Protein - Examples
• Whitefish • Wild salmon • White meat poultry • Shellfish • Lean red meat • Ostrich/Buffalo • Eggs • Cottage Cheese • Tempeh • Seitan	• Palm-sized serving • Low-fat • Organic • Nitrate-free • Non-allergenic • Omega-3 fats	• Cold cuts (preferably nitrate-free such as Boar's Head or Diestel brands) • Smoked salmon • Low-fat cheese • Precooked chicken • Shrimp cocktail • Hummus • Fat-free cream cheese • Low-fat or fat-free cottage cheese
High Fiber Starch - Best Sources	**High Fiber Starch - Concepts**	**Quick Starch - Examples**
• Oatmeal • Sweet potatoes • Brown rice • Whole grain pasta • Black beans • Split peas • Whole grain pita bread • Bulgur • Corn • Bran cereal • Popcorn • Pinto beans	• Unprocessed • Variety • Low sugar • Whole grain • Lower Glycemic Index	• Rye crisps • Sweet potatoes • Low-fat granola • Rye bread • Parboiled brown rice

Staples to pre-cook:	Produce to prep:
• Oatmeal	• Wash all
• Brown Rice	• Vacuum seal
• Whole grain noodles	• Dice melons
• Poultry	• Peel and freeze bananas
• Shrimp	• Dice onion
• Beans	
Meal Assembly Shopping List	**Healthy sauces:**
• Precooked chicken	• Pasta sauce
• Precooked rice	• Salsa
• Fresh pasta	• Stir fry
• Canned beans	• Vinaigrette
• Instant oatmeal	• EVOO/Balsamic vinegar
• Prepared lettuce	• BBQ
• Carrot sticks	• Thai peanut sauce
• Sliced mushrooms	• Curry
• Diced squash	• Tzatziki
• Baby bell peppers	• Hummus
• Baby spinach	• Mustard
• Veggies for dip	

GENERAL TIME SAVING TIPS:

• Shop for produce often - choose quick and easy
• Keep cooked staples on hand
• Keep sauces on hand
• Make extra supper for next day's lunch or snacks
• Shop perimeter of store

Shop for produce often and stock up on non-perishable items. Frozen fruit and vegetables are handy and very healthy. This way, if you need to stop by the supermarket during a busy week, it will just take a minute.

Keep cooked staples and pre-made sauces on hand. Sometimes life gets in the way and your available time to cook gets cut short or disappears all together. This will be easy to navigate when you already have what's needed to put together an easy and healthy meal at home.

Make extra food when you cook. If you take the time to plan and prepare a healthy meal, you might as well make it count. Pack away snack or lunch-size portions the same night. In the morning, just grab it and go!

A great tool when going to the supermarket is to remember to shop the perimeter of the store. This is where you'll find produce, meats, eggs, and dairy. Most everything found in the inner aisles is some mixture of wheat, sugar, salt and synthetic junk.

Snacks

Preparation is key when it comes to quality snacks. Measure and package snacks the night before a busy day, so you can just grab and go. Healthy snacking can keep your energy levels high and your mind alert.

- Nitrate- free cold cuts and high fiber crackers
- About 16-20 carrot sticks and two tablespoons of Tzatziki
- Cucumbers, tomatoes, and two tablespoons of hummus
- One medium apple and a small handful of nuts
- Two brown rice cakes with two ounces of smoked salmon, thin onion slices, and a dash of lemon juice
- One can of kippered snacks
- One medium pear

Breakfast

Huevos Rancheros
Layer:
1 corn tortilla
1/3 can fat-free refried beans
1 cup steamed spinach
2 eggs (poached, over easy or lightly basted)

Tip for Busy Mornings:
Hard-boil eggs in advance; it should take about 10 minutes to make enough eggs to last several days. After boiling the eggs, immerse in ice water. This will allow for easier shelling. Shell the eggs and refrigerate.

The morning of:
Prepare plate with tortilla on bottom, spread 1/3 small can refried beans and layer 2 cups of spinach leaves. Cover and microwave until spinach is wilted and tortilla and beans are warm. Optional toppings (for even more veggies) include diced tomatoes, 1/4 diced avocado, and 1/4 cup diced cilantro.

Ingredients: VegaPro™ protein powder (make sure the powder is without added sugar or flavorings), ground flaxseed, frozen berries

In a blender, place 1 serving VegaPro™ (1 scoop), 1-2 Tbs. of ground flax, and 1 cup of frozen berries. Add 1 cup water and blend.

Gourmet Oatmeal
Ingredients: Steel cut oats, natural sweetener (stevia or xylitol), cinnamon, nutmeg, Fiber One® cereal, coconut milk or unsweetened yogurt, apples

Tip for Busy Mornings:
Simmer 1 cup of steel cut oats for 30 minutes with 2 1/2 cups water. Add 1 tsp. natural sweetener, 1 tsp. cinnamon, and 1/8 tsp. nutmeg. For best results, use freshly grated nutmeg. This can all be done in advance; cooked oatmeal will keep for several days when refrigerated.

The morning of:
Warm up roughly 1/3 of the cooked oatmeal mixture. Add 1/4 cup Fiber One® cereal and 1/2 cup of either coconut milk or unsweetened yogurt. Top with 1/2 of an apple, diced.

Try amaranth cereal! It even sounds healthy, doesn't it? This wonderful grain is high in fiber, protein and calcium. Add 1 cup amaranth to 3 cups water and gently simmer for 30 minutes. This hot cereal has the most amazing texture and flavor. After cooking, sweeten like oatmeal and add 1 tsp. vanilla extract, 2 Tbs. sliced almonds, and 1/2 of a diced pear.

Lunch

Eating lunch out gives you poor quality food while wasting time and money. For most people, it's easier to eat a good evening meal consisting of protein, vegetables and a little starch. The most efficient way to have a good lunch is to pack it up the night before. Get in the habit of cooking more than you need for your evening meal and packing up a serving for the following day's lunch.

- Nitrate free cold cuts, sprouted bread, low fat cheese, veggies
- Split pea soup and an apple
- Rice noodles, shrimp, broccoli, and Better Than Bouillon brand vegetable stock

A great lunch example is the gourmet sandwich. Done well, the humble sandwich can be phenomenally tasty, healthy and quick.

Bread: If you're wheat sensitive, try Ezekiel® brand breads or use a corn tortilla and make your sandwich into wraps. If you're not wheat intolerant and have access to health food style supermarkets, try to find bread with just a few ingredients; the first should be whole wheat flour. If health food (specialty) supermarkets are inconvenient, try some of the brands with added fiber.

Meats: Cold cuts are handy and tasty but most contain nitrates. It's important to avoid nitrates; they raise your risk of stomach cancer. The other thing to consider when eating cold cuts is your total sodium intake over the day, because they do give you quite a bit. A better way to go is to use precooked poultry or meat from home that's sliced or shredded. If you're avoiding meat, consider egg salad. I like to use twice the number of whites as yolks. Smoked tofu or vegetarian 'cold cuts' are also great options for vegetarians or vegans.

Spreads: Nonfat cream cheese works great. To boost protein and fiber, think outside the box and try using hummus or refried black or pinto beans. Mustard is fine, as is mayo used sparingly or mixed with 1-2 parts of nonfat yogurt; this will lower the fat and raise the protein.

Veggies: The sky's the limit! So many taste great in sandwiches and they will boost your day's total servings. Lettuce is great, but don't waste your time on iceberg; get red leaf or romaine. Spinach also works well. Tomatoes are, of course, awesome antioxidants and an excellent addition to any sandwich. Sliced onions add zing, and an easy trick to prevent bad breath for your afternoon at work is to add some sprigs of fresh parsley. One fourth or 1/2 of an avocado tastes great and boosts fiber. Other good options include shaved carrot, sprouts, and sliced or roasted red bell pepper.

Pesto

Basil is known as an 'adaptogen.' This means it buffers the highs and lows of your adrenal and thyroid functions. It is also a great immune tonic. Try making this recipe when you're feeling frazzled or like you might get sick.

Pesto: This is a blended mix of a green herb, usually basil, but cilantro can work well in a pinch. Expect to use 2 ounces of fresh basil per person.

Starch: Linguini is the standby, but pesto works great on brown rice or Bulgur wheat. I especially like vegetable rotini with added fiber; it does a great job of holding onto the pesto. If you're wheat sensitive, try brown rice pastas or sliced and grilled polenta (cornmeal). If you are watching your weight, try Shirataki noodles. They cook fast, taste amazing, are gluten-free and net zero calories!

Protein: If you're in a rush, just serve some precooked chicken breast or cottage cheese alongside your pesto and starch. If you have time, try marinating poultry in garlic, basil, balsamic vinegar and olive oil. Expect it to look dark from the vinegar. Meat tends to be a bit heavy for the pesto.

For the meal, cook the starch and the protein and have them warm. When everyone is sitting down and ready, then it is time to make the pesto. It is at its peak of flavor for only moments after it is blended. It can be as simple as putting lightly washed basil in the blender, stems removed. Add 2 tsp. lemon juice and just enough olive oil to blend. You can also include 1/3 cup lightly toasted pine nuts, 1/2 cup feta cheese (try fat free, it tastes the same!), 1-2 cloves of garlic and a pinch of cayenne pepper.

Burrito Bowl

- Grilled chicken
- Precooked brown rice
- Precooked black beans
- Fresh salsa (recipe below)

In a bowl, add ½ cup brown rice and about a handful of chicken. Layer a ½ cup of black beans on top with fresh tomato salsa.

Fresh Tomato Salsa

- Tomatoes
- Onion
- Cilantro
- Jalapenos
- Green onion
- Garlic powder
- Salt and pepper

Combine about 3 chopped tomatoes with half a diced onion. Stir in a handful of cilantro leaves and ¼ cup of chopped jalapenos and green onions. Season to taste with garlic powder and salt and pepper.

Dinner

Stir Fry

Ingredients:
Precooked brown rice
Mixed stir fry veggies (can find these already chopped, either fresh or frozen)
Precooked white meat chicken breast (can also find this fresh or frozen)
Teriyaki sauce
Toasted sesame oil

The prep could not be easier. Sauté the veggies in 1-2 tsp. of toasted sesame oil, and add diced chicken, 2 sheets of crumbled nori and sauce. Serve over warmed rice.

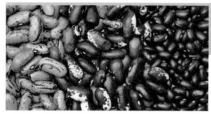

Beans

By Dr. Alan Christianson

Beans and legumes are the richest sources of all types of fiber available. They are also high in crucial nutrients like folate and magnesium. For some, they can be hard to digest without getting lots of gas. What happens is that the fibers in beans encourage the growth of certain strains of bacteria called Bifidobacterium. If you are low in these bacteria, the sudden growth will mean lots of methane is formed, leading to uncomfortable gas. If you know you are sensitive to this reaction, the solution is not to avoid beans, but to introduce them into your diet slowly. Try just 1-2 Tbs. black beans each day for two weeks. In most cases, this causes a gentle shift in the bacteria, which is mild enough not to cause discomfort, but strong enough to allow you to tolerate all the beans you like after these first two weeks.

The other consideration about beans is cooking. Dry beans cook best when sorted, soaked overnight, rinsed, boiled for a few hours and stored. Most bags of dry beans are at least a pound. If you take the time to go through this, you will have a large batch, which has a short shelf life. Canned foods in general are good to avoid, but canned beans are fine. Look for brands that have no ingredients other than beans, water and possibly salt. Choose salt-free or lower-salt versions. Look for under 150 milligrams of sodium per serving.

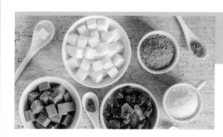

Sweeteners

By Dr. Alan Christianson

Sugar is unhealthy, but are artificial sweeteners better? Evidence is growing that artificially sweetened foods lead to weight gain. Which sweeteners are best to use? The main issues to look at include whether it is toxic, how many calories it has, how much fructose it has, how much it affects our blood sugar and whether it suppresses the immune system. Once we apply all of these filters, not too many are left. Sugar, brown sugar, molasses, raw sugar and turbinado sugar do badly on all counts. Sucralose (Splenda®) and aspartame (NutraSweet®) can be toxic and disrupt our blood sugar. Agave nectar, honey and coconut sugar are high in fructose, which is hard on the liver and causes the most weight gain.

Stevia and Monk Fruit (Lo Han) are plant extracts that have a sweet taste but no calories. Both have been thoroughly studied and shown to be safe. They may even have some antioxidants and help blood sugar. The one drawback is that they can taste bitter. Your best option is to buy a few different brands of pure stevia and monk fruit and see which one tastes the best to you.

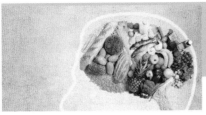

Being Mindful of How You Eat

By Dr. Adrienne Stewart

Being mindful is about allowing our consciousness to rest fully on what we are doing in the moment. We are constantly bombarded by information, so it is easy to become distracted and disconnected from the present. When this happens, we make choices unconsciously that aren't always in our best interest, such as grabbing a candy bar for a snack. When we become more aware of what and how we are eating, we start making healthier choices that will empower our lives and our health.

Mindful eating also helps us:

Recognize when we are full before we overeat.

Savor the flavors and textures of the foods we are eating.

Calm our parasympathetic system for improved digestion.

Make better food choices.

Mindful eating includes all aspects of preparing food – from shopping to cooking to eating.

Mindful Shopping

Many of our healthiest choices begin with where and how we shop. While many stores are carrying organic groceries, it is also a good idea to support local farmers' markets. They provide fresh, seasonal, organic foods, plus you are supporting the local economy. When considering organic food options, it is a great idea to start with organic meat and produce. The Environmental Working Group publishes the *Dirty Dozen Plus*™, a list of produce that has the highest exposure to pesticides. These twelve foods are best to buy organic. Then, their list of the *Clean Fifteen*™ names the foods lowest in pesticides, which are not as essential to buy organic. For buying meat, look for grass-fed, grass-finished, free range, and organic meats. For fish, try wild-caught. Another helpful tip is to shop the perimeter of the grocery store. This is where you will find fresh whole foods rather than the highly-processed boxed and canned foods in the center aisles.

If you have food sensitivities, learn where to find your gluten-free, dairy-free and vegan options. Experiment with different brands and recipes to find what you like. Also, focus on changing bad habits by not buying foods and candy that you don't want around the house. Replace these foods with healthy snacks that you can grab on the go. If the food is available, it will more likely be eaten. So, make those healthy choices in the store.

Mindful Cooking

Meal planning is an excellent way to bring mindfulness to cooking. Set time aside for meal preparation by planning the night before, preparing meals during the weekend, or using Crockpot recipes. These are all easy ways to prepare healthy meals for the entire family. One of the most important aspects of mindful cooking is to engage in the present moment with the food you prepare; try new recipes, experiment with new spices, and remember to have fun. By cooking, smelling, and being mindful of food, you help stimulate digestive enzymes that start digestion before you take your first bite.

Mindful Cooking

Meal planning is an excellent way to bring mindfulness to cooking.

Remember to be mindful of your snack choices as well. Preparing healthy snacks in advance can help you avoid reaching for a quick fix that you may regret later. Spend some time washing and chopping veggie sticks so they are ready to go in the refrigerator. Another way to avoid unhealthy snacks is to eat before you become famished. If you eat regular meals throughout the day, you balance your blood sugar and are less likely to binge when hunger pushes you over the edge.

Mindful Eating

When you do sit down to enjoy your meal, try engaging all your senses. Become aware of the textures, smells, colors and taste of your food. Also, become aware of your body while you eat. Notice when your hunger is satiated, and stop when you feel full rather than when your plate is empty.

One of the most important aspects of mindful eating is to focus on the process rather than multitasking. Avoid watching TV, doing work, or checking email while eating to avoid unconscious food choices. One way to do this is to set the table and eat as a family, taking the time to relax, connect, and talk about the day.

Make sure to chew and breathe with a steady, moderate pace. Chewing improves digestion and breathing helps relax your nervous system. You might try setting your fork down between bites to help slow down the processes.

Gratitude is an important aspect of mindful eating, whether you prefer to say a prayer or simply give thanks. Make sure to consciously send gratitude to everyone who helped bring the food to your table - the farmers who grew the food, the grocery store employees who worked to keep the food fresh, and yourself for cooking and preparing such a healthy meal for you and your family.

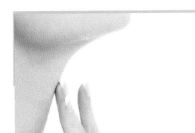

Thyroid-Specific Nutrients

By Dr. Alan Christianson

With hypothyroidism, you have nutritional requirements that are distinct from everyone else. Many common recommendations that are made for the general population are not appropriate or helpful for you. Some nutrients are best for you to avoid, while some are even more important for you than they are for others. These same concerns hold true about various foods. To clear the air and avoid confusion, I have streamlined all of the basic nutrient guidelines to support thyroid health.

The best strategies for you are straightforward and easy to act on.

IODINE
Iodine is the center of it all when it comes to thyroid health. Most other nutrients are only important because they assist or detract from iodine.

The funny thing about iodine is that we get it in our salt, and we get too much salt, yet some people can be low in iodine. How can this be? Nearly all Americans consume sodium well in excess of 2500 mg daily and, since processed foods are made with non-iodized salt, patients should be advised to minimize their salt intake from restaurant foods and pre-made groceries. Instead, their prime sodium intake should be from home cooked foods made with conservative use of iodized table salt or iodized sea salt.

Along with iodized salt, consuming a variety of fruits, vegetables, meats, seafood and grains can provide a basal amount of iodine. Additionally, pregnant and lactating women should be advised to consume a multivitamin containing 50-100 mcgs of iodine daily.

Keep it Simple
You do need some iodine in your diet, but too much is dangerous. If you are on a thyroid replacement, you are already taking an iodine pill.

Food Sources

The best choices for iodine-rich foods include low-fat dairy, bread, fresh produce, seafood, and iodized salt or sea salt.

Selenium

Selenium prevents free radical damage to the thyroid, aids in iodine absorption and helps the body utilize thyroid hormones.

SELENIUM

Iodine's sidekick, Selenium, is needed to protect the thyroid against free radical damage. It eliminates toxins that hurt the thyroid and helps activate thyroid hormones after they are formed. 200 – 400 mcgs should be consumed daily through your diet and supplements.

Keep It Simple

Selenium prevents free radical damage to the thyroid, aids in iodine absorption and helps the body utilize thyroid hormones.

Food Sources

The richest food source of selenium by far is the Brazil nut. Eating only one per day can give you all the selenium you need, but if you get too much it can be toxic. Be careful not to average more than 10 per week. Selenium can also be found in brown rice and chia seeds.

ZINC

Zinc is needed for the chemical conversion of iodine within the thyroid. There are a few reasons that people don't get the zinc they need. First, most diets high in processed foods are often low in zinc. Secondly, it's a rather hard mineral to absorb. And lastly, people with digestive issues may have problems absorbing zinc, even if they eat enough.

Keep It Simple

Staying away from processed foods allows your body to use zinc for optimal thyroid function.

Food Sources

If you like oysters, you're in luck! Oysters are to zinc what Brazil nuts are to selenium. Other good sources include meat, fish and wheat germ.

VITAMIN A

Vitamin A is needed for proper intake of iodine into the thyroid. It's also important to know that if there is too little Vitamin A in the body, the thyroid can form goiters or nodules. Healthy people can make Vitamin A from Beta-carotene in their diets. Paradoxically, it can be hard for people who have thyroid disease to make this conversion.

Keep It Simple

Keeping adequate Vitamin A levels in the body can help ward off the formation of goiters or nodules.

Food Sources

Not sure how well your body does with making Beta-carotene from Vitamin A? No need to worry. You can get it directly from eggs, herring, tuna and salmon.

IRON

If iron levels are low, it raises the risk of developing a goiter. It can also compound fatigue symptoms that come from hypothyroidism. One common culprit for a low iron level is regular blood loss. This is quite relevant when you consider that the majority of those with thyroid disease are women and many are diagnosed while in their menstruating years. Keep in mind that iron level testing is important, since it can be toxic if too much is consumed. On your blood tests, look for the ideal iron range of 65 – 100 mcg/L.

> ## Iron
> The ideal range for iron in your blood is 65-100 mcg/L. Be mindful of your levels and adjust your diet as necessary

Keep It Simple

The ideal range for iron in your blood is 65 – 100 mcg/L. Be mindful of your levels and adjust your diet as necessary.

Food Sources

The best food sources are red meat, dark meat poultry and egg yolks. You can also get iron from plant sources like spinach. While these plants are healthy foods, they contain non-heme iron, which is poorly absorbed.

GOITROGENS

A goiter is an enlargement of the thyroid. In the modern world, it's most commonly caused by autoimmune disease. However, it can also be triggered by certain chemicals. These chemicals are called goitrogens as a group, even though they work in very different ways. Some of them are naturally occurring in foods. If you've read about thyroid diets before, you may have seen a list of possible goitrogenic foods.

It can be difficult to understand the difference between chemical types of goitrogens. Some really are worth avoiding and some are not.

The other problem is that some foods actually have been observed to be goitrogenic, while the vast majority are classified that way only by theory.

This means their effects have never been observed in a human. They are simply thought to be goitrogenic due to their chemical effects on animals.

In many cases, goitrogens have no relevant impact on those with thyroid disease. When they are found in vegetables, they have a very weak effect on inhibiting iodine absorption. These chemicals are also very fragile and destroyed by cooking. That being said, there are rare instances when goitrogens in vegetables are a concern. For example, if someone consumes many pounds of raw broccoli daily and does not consume adequate amounts of iodized salt, dairy, seafood or sea vegetables. This person may want to be concerned with goitrogens. The lack of certain nutrients can trigger goiters as well as consuming excess amounts of goitrogens.

Let me give you a more practical example. 'Jake' was a previously healthy young man who was brought to my practice by his father, who was concerned that he was getting apathetic and weak. Several months earlier, Jake had embarked on a 100% raw produce diet. He was very passionate about the diet and the benefits he felt it was providing him. His meals consisted mostly of blended raw vegetables with small amounts of fruit. This made it easy for him to consume 3 – 5 pounds of broccoli a day. We ran a few tests and found that Jake had iron and B-12 deficiency anemia. Along with this, he had hypothyroidism with no apparent signs of an autoimmune response. Luckily, Jake was willing to make a few concessions. I admired his efforts to take charge of his health and go off the beaten path. In honoring that, I only asked him to make a few changes. He added back into his diet low mercury fish and sea vegetables and, in doing so, avoided the extreme amounts of raw cruciferous vegetables. I also asked him to be mindful of his consumption of soy foods and millet, as these foods are relevant goitrogens. This plan allowed him to stay on track with his passion for better health and, within a few months, he had normal thyroid function again. Unless you are in Jake's situation, you can be sure that there is much more to gain by eating vegetables than by avoiding them.

Keep It Simple
Eat your broccoli, spinach and kale while minimizing soy foods and millet.

PROTEIN
Since thyroid disease causes a slowing of metabolic rate, getting adequate protein without getting too many calories is the key to staying lean. Protein is an important part of each cell in the body, so it makes sense that protein is essential in our diet.

The best options for protein are the ones that are low in fat and minimally processed. Occasionally, it's alright to have red meat – just try to cut out the fat because that's where the toxins are concentrated. When it comes to choosing your protein, wild and organic are best to avoid pesticides, antibiotics, and other contaminants. Milk, yogurt, and cheese are not great protein options since they provide more carbohydrate, sugar, and fat calories than they do protein calories. An appropriate portion of protein should be about the size of your palm.

Keep it Simple
Focus on lean proteins from good sources and keep your portions appropriate.

Food Sources
Good examples of lean protein are salmon, white meat poultry, and shellfish. Eggs are a good source of protein as well. For all the vegetarians and vegans out there, try tempeh, hummus, and other meat alternatives.

FOOD INTOLERANCES
People with an autoimmune disorder like thyroid disease are more likely to have food intolerances, and their reactions tend to be more severe. Typical foods that can cause such reactions include peanuts, shellfish and berries. Most commonly, these foods do nothing in the moment, but will gradually increase inflammation and aggravate digestive symptoms.

Those with thyroid disease should undergo screening for these reactions at least once a year. This can be done with a simple home test kit or can be done in the doctor's office by a blood draw. Skin allergy tests are available and accurate for quick onset allergies. However, they do not reveal delayed onset reactions. The other option is to do an elimination diet. In this process, a non-allergenic meal substitute is used with a few simple foods for several days. Then, foods are introduced slowly while symptoms are monitored.

Food Intolerances

People with an autoimmune disorder like thyroid disease are more likely to have food intolerances, and their reactions tend to be more severe.

BLOOD SUGAR CONTROL
Many people with thyroid disease have poor regulation of blood sugar. This can cause diabetes, fatty liver, weight gain, fatigue, and mood changes. Control of blood sugar is achieved by structuring your diet carefully. The main considerations are when you eat, what you eat, and what you don't eat.

When to Eat

It's very important to start the day with a solid breakfast. If you are short on time, try a shake or a Control Bar. Mid-morning, have a light snack, then plan on having an earlier lunch. You can add a mid-afternoon snack if you need it, but always make it a point to have a light dinner and stop eating by 7 pm. You sleep best when you're not famished, but just a little hungry. This also makes it easier to lose weight.

What not to eat

The foods that throw off your blood sugar the most are those that have more than 5 grams of sugar per serving, or more than 1/3 of their calories from fat. Sugar grams per serving are easy to find, as they are on the food label. Percent of fat calories can be found by looking at total calories and fat grams. Fat is roughly 10 calories per gram. So, you simply multiply fat grams by 10, then divide this number into the total calories. For example, say a serving of potato chips has 300 calories and 15 grams of fat per serving. Take 15 (total fat grams) and multiply it by 10 to get 150. You then take 300 (total calories) and divide it by 150, giving you 50%, meaning half of their calories are from fat.

Hopefully, it is not a surprise to learn that potato chips are not a good food. Did you know they are the densest known source of calories by weight? Climbers on high alpine mountains lose weight due to the extreme conditions. They also need to minimize the weight of their packs. For these reasons, one of their most practical foods is crushed potato chips. If you really want to enjoy them guilt free, be sure to sign up for an Everest expedition!

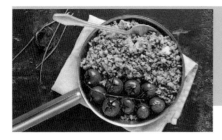

Gluten-Free Tips for Patients with Thyroid Disease

By Dr. Adrienne Stewart

Diet is an important factor in managing chronic health conditions like thyroid disease, because certain nutrients affect how well the thyroid gland functions. Gluten-free diets are often recommended for people with thyroid disease because gluten, the protein found in wheat and other types of grains, is a common allergen that may trigger inflammation in the body and exacerbate autoimmune conditions like Hashimoto's Thyroiditis and Graves' disease. Research has shown a strong correlation between Celiac disease, which is an aggressive autoimmune response to gluten, and other autoimmune diseases. For those with Celiac disease, gluten can damage the lining of the small intestine and prevent the body from absorbing nutrients properly.

There are other kinds of immune responses to gluten in addition to Celiac disease that can aggravate thyroid health. IgG immune responses to gluten are delayed hypersensitivity reactions, with symptoms often developing hours to days after ingesting the offending food. This type of immune response is called food sensitivity. Food sensitivities can manifest as difficulty maintaining stable thyroid levels, weight gain or weight loss resistance, chronic inflammation in joints, digestive issues such as diarrhea, gas, and bloating, and even damage to the digestive tract. This can make it difficult to assimilate nutrients from food, which often leads to fatigue. Repeated intake of a food sensitivity often leads to other food sensitivities and can even trigger autoimmune conditions. It is important to test for gluten sensitivity by running a simple IgG Food Allergy Test with the help of your naturopathic doctor.

Many health professionals recommend gluten-free diets for everyone, regardless if someone has a direct sensitivity or not. Gluten-free diets encourage us to replace gluten sources such as wheat, barley, and rye with other nutrient-rich grains like amaranth and quinoa. Health is always improved when we can get more nutrition into the diet, especially through food sources. Gluten-free diets also tend to lower the amount of highly processed carbohydrates we consume, which leaves room for more nutritious choices such as fruits, vegetables, and lean proteins.

Considering its many health benefits, here are some tips for going gluten-free:

1. **Read Labels.** Going gluten-free can be challenging in a traditional Western diet because many processed foods contain hidden sources of gluten. For example, you might find gluten in condiments like soy sauce or in canned foods, like soups. You might even find it in your ice cream. Gluten-free diets often require you to read food labels carefully. It is important to keep in mind that gluten is in many grains, but not in all. There are nutritious and delicious alternatives. The Celiac Support Association has one of the most comprehensive resources on gluten-free grains (http://www.csaceliacs.info/grains_and_flours_glossary.jsp). This can help when reading food labels. The good news is that more companies are now indicating if something is gluten-free and including lists of common food allergens on their product labels.

Read labels

Going gluten-free can be challenging in a traditional Western diet because many processed foods contain hidden sources of gluten. For example, you might find gluten in condiments like soy sauce or in canned foods, like soups.

2. **Food Substitutions.** In addition to better food labels, companies are also making gluten-free alternatives for common products like cereals and breads. It is even possible to find gluten-free baking mixes that taste wonderful. Shopping at your local health food store or farmers' market is an important part of a gluten-free lifestyle. Creative food substitutions can often make going gluten-free barely noticeable. For example, brown rice flour tortillas or corn tortillas are often a great replacement for flour tortillas. Be sure to read the food labels to make sure it is truly gluten-free. An even healthier alternative would be lettuce wraps, which are crisp, healthy, and carb-free. Another great food substitution is rice noodles or spaghetti squash in place of pasta. Many of the common foods we love can be substituted for gluten-free alternatives that taste good and are nutritious.

3. **Home Cooking.** The easiest way to know if a meal is gluten-free is to make it yourself. Many popular recipe sites now have sections for gluten-free recipes. There are also many gluten-free cookbooks, many of which can be found in your local health food store. Most gluten-containing flours can be substituted for bean flours, nut flours, and other gluten-free grains. It often requires a mix of several types of flour to get the consistency that we are used to in wheat bread. Homemade food can also be very nutritious, especially if you are following a whole foods diet that is full of fruits, vegetables, and lean protein.

Although going gluten-free can be challenging for families, especially those with picky eaters, it comes with many health benefits. For those with thyroid disease, it is especially important to investigate the possibility of gluten sensitivity with your doctor. As awareness about gluten allergies grow, so do the resources and support for embracing a gluten-free lifestyle.

Gluten-Free Chocolate Chip Walnut Cookies

Ingredients:

1 C. sunflower seed flour (must be finely ground - a high speed blender works best)
2 Tbs. coconut flour, sifted
3/4 C. tapioca starch
1 tsp. baking powder
1/4 C. cocoa powder
1/4 tsp. sea salt

1/4 C. pure maple syrup
2 tsp. pure vanilla extract
2 Tbs. applesauce
2 Tbs. coconut oil, melted
1/4 C. gluten-free dark chocolate chips
1/4 cup walnuts

Instructions:
1. Preheat oven to 350°.
2. In a medium bowl, add dry ingredients (sunflower seed flour, coconut flour, tapioca starch, baking powder, cocoa powder, sea salt). Stir to combine.
3. Add wet ingredients to the dry (maple syrup, vanilla extract, applesauce, coconut oil). Blend with a hand mixer until fully combined. Stir in chocolate chips and walnuts.
4. Scoop by rounded tablespoons of dough onto a parchment-lined baking sheet. This dough doesn't spread while baking, so flatten with a fork before baking.
5. Bake 11-13 minutes or until edges are set and center is slightly firm to the touch. Cool on trays on wire racks for 5 minutes. Remove cookies to wire racks to cool completely. Store in an airtight container for up to 4 days, or freeze until needed.

Who Needs Iodine?

By Dr. Alan Christianson

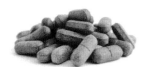

Since the nuclear reactor disaster in Japan, countless people have been taking iodine supplements. Many have just been stockpiling against possible need, but a sizable number have been taking megadoses of iodine prophylactically. All scientific sources have stated that those in the continental United States have no significant risks whatsoever from the events in Japan. Nonetheless, people are taking iodine out of panic.

Unfortunately, taking iodine at the wrong time guarantees it won't work if it really is needed. Furthermore, 8-10% of the population has latent thyroid problems, making them prone to serious side effects from iodine pills.

Adults over 40 are most at risk for iodine side effects and have no clear benefit from using preventive iodine. Many are taking it daily, creating no possible benefit, and increasing their risk for substantial side effects, including stroke and heart attack.

Our thyroid glands depend on iodine to work properly. Since they so aggressively concentrate iodine, they are at risk to concentrate radioactive iodine in the event of nuclear fallout. History has shown that those exposed to low levels of radiation faced much higher rates of eventual thyroid cancer. Since thyroid cancer takes decades to form, this risk is highest in neonates, infants, children and adolescents, in that order. Adults under 40 have very minimal risk of thyroid cancer secondary to radiation exposure, yet their risk from iodine per protocol is also low. Adults over 40 face much more risk of iodine side effects than they do benefit, even with significant, local exposure.

The rationale of iodine-loading supplements is that when the thyroid gland is completely full of iodine, it quits absorbing it for a period of time, making it less vulnerable to storing radioactive iodine.

Potassium iodide, which supplies 65% iodine, can protect against radioactive iodine, but not other radioactive elements, for a 24-hour window.

When needed, iodine is best given in a single dose, ideally 4-24 hours prior to exposure.

The following are dosing instructions per the post-Chernobyl World Health Organization Protocol:

Age group	Single dose of iodine (mg)	Fraction of 100 mg tablet
12-39	100	1
3-12	50	1/2
1 month – 3 years	25	1/4
Birth – 1 month	12.5	1/8

People should not take iodine if they have:
• History of thyroid disease
• Active thyroid antibodies
• History of iodine allergy
• Dermatitis herpetiformis

The complicating factor is that many without a known history of thyroid disease do have active thyroid antibodies.

Megadose iodine has also become a fad in the natural health community. Here is some more information I've written about the dangers of this practice:

Iodine. Not too much, not too little.

In Arizona, many retirees spend their summers elsewhere. To me, it marks the change of seasons to welcome my 'snowbirds' back in the fall and see them off in the spring.

Several years ago, I had a kind gentleman return for the winter with new symptoms: watery diarrhea after every meal and a non-intentional tremor of his hand. The diarrhea had started three or four months previously, the tremor, more recently. Normally in excellent health, 'Tim' joked about getting old and his body falling apart. He had his screening tests completed before I heard about this. They were normal besides a suppressed TSH. On his exam, I found several thyroid nodules that were not present last year, and his heart rate was over 100 bpm.

An ultrasound and second-level thyroid tests diagnosed Tim with toxic multinodular goiter. In seniors, this is most common after high dose iodine exposure, such as in imaging contrast. I asked if he had a CT or MRI done recently. He told me he did not but that he was taking an iodine pill for five months. Apparently he was tested and found to be low in iodine and was now taking 1 tablet of Iodoral daily, providing 50,000 mcg of iodine.

Within several months, I had roughly the same thing happen to three other patients. All were on high dose iodine, some based on testing, some not. One of these also had toxic multinodular goiter, one had Graves' disease, and one was hypothyroid secondary to Hashimoto's Thyroiditis. Since then, several more cases have come in with new thyroid disease after taking high dose iodine.

Not all patients who take high dose iodine will get thyroid disease, and it is possible that some that I saw may have developed thyroid disease even if not on iodine. I have seen many other patients taking high dose iodine with no apparent adverse effects.

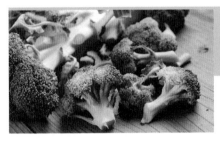

Clearing Up Some Common Myths

By Dr. Alan Christianson

Does Broccoli Hurt Your Thyroid? If you eat three-plus pounds of broccoli raw daily and you're iodine deficient, yes. If you have thyroid disease and are on treatment, no.

Lots of data shows that broccoli can cut the risk of many cancers, including thyroid cancers. This is also true of many healthy vegetables that find their way on the lists of 'goitrogens.' Without perspective on what a goitrogen is or what it does, it would be easy to feel compelled to avoid many healthy foods for fear of harming the thyroid. Goitrogens are not specific chemicals, but rather a large category of chemicals with completely different effects on thyroid function, some more relevant than others.

Genistein, from soy, is one of the few things that can affect the course of autoimmune thyroid disease. Nearly all other goitrogens act by slowing iodine absorption into the thyroid. In parts of the world like sub-Saharan Africa, for example, some populations are on the edge of iodine deficiency. If a population like this consumes high amounts of cassava, they may worsen the iodine deficiency.

The main chemicals in foods that affect this are indole compounds. These are also known to lower the risk of many cancers, including thyroid cancer. People with thyroid disease have a higher risk for thyroid cancer.

Most thyroid disease in the modern world is caused by autoimmune disease, as opposed to iodine deficiency. Furthermore, thyroid treatment medicines all contain iodine. Because of this, the possible small impairment of iodine absorption from goitrogens is smaller than the health benefits, and cooking goitrogens eliminates this consideration altogether.

What are the best action steps?
• Make sure you're on the best dose of thyroid medicine
• If you've never had a thyroid ultrasound, get one done as a baseline
• Have your broccoli in good health and enjoy it
• Avoid high amounts of soy

Is wine a health food?

Is wine a health food?

You may have heard that small amounts may be mildly protective for your heart. Unfortunately, data is now getting stronger that any amount of alcohol from any source, including wine, damages the brain. In a study of 1839 brain scans, researchers showed that brain shrinkage was exactly related to alcohol intake and there was no amount that caused no shrinkage. Dr. Daniel Amen tells us, when it comes to the brain, size does matter. If wine is an important part of your life, try 6 weeks without it. This is good to do at least once per year. Much of the gradual damage of alcohol is worse when our body never has a break from it. If this idea makes you uncomfortable, ask yourself what it is about wine that you would miss the most for 6 weeks – the taste? Could you avoid your favorite vegetable for 6 weeks? Sure, this would not be a big deal. You might be surprised how much your sleep quality, daily energy levels, and brain function improve. If nothing obvious happens, your brain will still thank you, and you can always go right back to drinking your wine.

No, red meat does not cause cancer

The research behind *The China Study* showed animal protein did not raise the risk of cancer, even though the authors of it and the movie *Forks Over Knives* alleged that it did. In the post, I mentioned that large studies have not yet separated vegetarianism from healthy lifestyles. In general, vegetarians are leaner, less likely to smoke and tend to eat more produce than those without intentional diets. I also argued that if lean, non-smoking, produce eating non-vegetarians were compared against vegetarians, there would not be a benefit.

This was a huge study of 511,781 people in 23 countries. The main question it set out to answer was this: if you take out other important variables such as smoking, body weight, physical activity, alcohol intake and produce intake, does red meat, poultry or processed meat cause cancer?

A recent US study looked at this topic, but failed to differentiate red meat from processed meat. Processed meat is defined as smoked or cured meat such as sausage, bacon or lunch meat. Numerous prior studies have shown the nitrate-based preservatives in it are carcinogenic.

What were the results from the most powerful and well-designed study to date? Red meat does not cause cancer, nor does poultry. Unsurprisingly, processed meat does. To be healthy you do want to exercise, don't smoke, limit alcohol, consume lots of produce and avoid processed food, including processed meat. Adding fish, poultry and red meat (especially grass fed) will supply more bone and muscle-building protein and other essential nutrients. Animal protein is part of a healthy lifestyle.

Do you really need to eat greens?

You hear the advice to eat leafy green vegetables all the time, but do they really matter? The most common reasons for eating them include fiber and folic acid. Greens don't really have that much fiber, and folic acid is fortified in even the unhealthiest of foods. One serving of spinach has no more fiber than popcorn and less than 1/4 the fiber of a serving of black beans. It also has the same amount of folic acid as Wonder® bread. So what's the big deal? Oftentimes, the advice to eat them is sound but the advisors are unclear on the real mechanism of benefit. Studies have shown repeatedly that diets higher in greens lower the risk of many types of cancer, including breast, lung, colorectal and prostate.

Many think the benefit comes from the benefit greens have on our body's detoxification mechanisms. We ingest many chemical wastes from our diet, our air and from our skin. We also make many wastes inside our bodies as a byproduct of forming energy, similar to the way a car makes exhaust.

The majority of these wastes are processed by our liver. After the liver does its thing, these wastes are sent to our intestinal tract to be carried out with our stool. Here's the problem: many modern chemicals that are in our stool on their way out, actually seep back into our blood stream in the colon.

The name for this is enterohepatic recirculation. This means our intestines recirculate things back to our liver. Sometimes this is helpful, like in the case of bile acids or cholesterol. Yet for many modern chemicals like pesticides, solvents and toxic metals, this means they may recirculate in our bodies so long, they never really get out.

What is the remedy for this? Remember Kermit the frog saying, "It isn't easy being green?" In the case of your poop and the chemicals in your body, remember it IS easy being green. The more pigment from green foods that finds its way to your stool, the more wastes leave for good. With green foods, more is better. Focus most on frequency. A little bit of spinach with several meals will give you more benefit than a larger amount less often. That's the real reason to eat greens.

The Truth on Diet Sodas

What is so bad about diet soda? Artificial sweeteners are worth avoiding, but not for the reasons you might think. First we had saccharine (Sweet 'N Low®), a known carcinogen. Then came aspartame (NutraSweet®). It is known to be toxic to brain cells. These are important to many of us. Newest is sucralose (Splenda®). Most soda manufacturers have switched to it.

Artificial sweeteners are worth avoiding, but not for the reasons you might think.

Many voiced concerns that the sweet taste alone altered blood sugar. After reading the studies, I was not convinced this was a big factor. Some studies showed it did happen to a tiny degree, and some showed it did not happen at all. Splenda® is also unique in that it is not absorbed. This means you taste it, swallow it and then poop it. It does not get into your blood stream and go through your brain, liver, kidneys – nothing. Now we have data saying it is harmful but for entirely different reasons. It turns out Splenda® kills your protective bacteria like antibiotics do. Among many other bad effects, the loss of some strains of good bacteria can actually make you fat! Do avoid artificial sweeteners. Two natural sweeteners that are okay to use, and even beneficial, include xylitol and stevia.

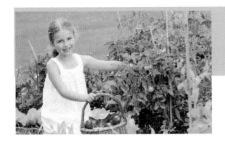

Fresh from the Garden

by Dr. Linda Khoshaba

Have you ever been told that when you eat any meal, it should resemble the colors of a rainbow? Well if not, now is your time to learn about how the color of fruits or vegetables can dramatically influence your health. Each fruit or vegetable has a unique color and function. Having a wide variety of colors in your meals can help you intake the necessary vitamins, minerals, antioxidants and phytochemicals that help with a balanced diet.

Although you can supplement with specific vitamins or minerals, eating your fruits and vegetables together creates a synergistic effect and yields the maximum amount of health benefits. Here is a breakdown of the rainbow spectrum of foods, and what benefits you can achieve by simply adding them to your meals at least once a day.

Dark Cruciferous Greens
Cruciferous vegetables are rich sources of sulphur-containing compounds known as glucosinolates. The taste of them is often described as pungent, bitter or spicy. These types of vegetables include kale, bok choy, spinach, arugula, and broccoli, and are especially important in helping detoxify your body. Detoxification is a process your liver undergoes to help you neutralize and eliminate the chemical wastes and byproducts you produce each day. There are two main phases of detoxification. Phase 1 consists of processing chemicals to make them ready for Phase 2. Phase 2 is where you excrete the toxins from your body. These types of vegetables contain sulphoraphane, an indirect antioxidant, which acts to induce Phase 2 detoxification. Other benefits of sulphoraphane include tumor inhibition and systemic anti-inflammatory effects.

Greens
Vegetables in this color spectrum contain phytochemicals known as lutein and indoles. Lutein, part of the carotenoid family, is a powerful antioxidant that is essential for vision. Indole has been known for its powerful anti-carcinogenic effects. Look for foods such as avocados, artichokes, green cabbage, celery, lettuce and peas. Common garden herbs such as thyme, basil, sage and mint are also full of phytochemicals. These herbs not only add flavor and freshen the taste of your meal, they can be used as a substitute for salt, sugar and fat in any meal.

Reds

Lycopene and anthocyanins are the two most common constituents found in red-colored fruits and vegetables. Lycopenes are carotenoids known for antioxidant and anti-proliferative effects. Tomatoes, guava, apricots and watermelon are well known for their lycopene content. The bioavailabity of lycopene is highest in cooked and pureed tomatoes, and this is a common dietary recommendation given to men with prostate conditions. Anthocyanins are flavonoids, known for the pigment found in foods such as berries, pomegranates, red onions, and kidney beans. These pigments boost your overall health and exert their antioxidant effects throughout your entire body.

Oranges

When you see the color orange, no doubt the first thing you think about is either a sour citrus flavor or Vitamin C. But those are not the only things orange should have a reputation for. Orange-colored fruits and vegetables have a number of other benefits ranging from heart to immune health. Beta-carotene, a form of Vitamin A, has strong antiviral properties and increases immune function by increasing the number of T lymphocytes. Satisfy a sweet craving by making a quick and easy fruit salad with fruits such as grapefruit, peaches, papaya, tangerines, mangos, and cantaloupe!

Yellow

Representing joy and happiness, this may be related to the way these fruits & vegetables taste.

Yellows

You will see some overlap of similar actions between the yellow and orange foods. Yellow is a unique color that represents joy and happiness, and may be related to the way these fruits and vegetables taste. Lemons, bananas, golden delicious apples, yellow peppers, corn, pineapples and squash are excellent in reducing inflammation, stimulating wound healing and contain properties that strengthen your teeth and bones.

Blues/Purples

You may think that adding blue/purple fruits or vegetables to a daily meal is challenging, but it can be as simple as throwing some blueberries, blackberries, plums or raisins into a breakfast meal. This color group is specifically known for lutein, zeaxanthin, quercetin and resveratrol components. Zeaxanthin has been studied for its effects on vision and how it helps prevent age-related macular degeneration. Quercetin, another type of flavonoid, not only is anti-inflammatory, but also has some blood pressure lowering effects.

As you can see, there are endless benefits to eating a wide variety of foods. The color represents a small clue as to the role of that particular food. So, get started and have fun coloring your rainbow!

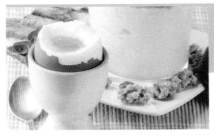

Adrenals and Blood Sugar

By Dr. Alan Christianson

Secret formula to be happy and lean: 70-100 mg/dl.

That's it. That's the secret formula.

Okay, here's some more detail. The numbers refer to the ideal ranges of your blood sugar.

When there is too little, your brain and muscles can't work at their best. When there is too much, even for a few minutes, lots of bad things happen.

Your blood cells are little discs that rush around in your blood vessels. They leave the blood vessels through tiny openings and bring badly needed oxygen to your body.

When your blood sugar gets too high, sugar sticks to the outside of these cells. Have you ever used a misting bottle with water for your plants or your hair? How well would maple syrup work in that bottle? How well would corn syrup work in that bottle if it had been sitting for a week?

That is exactly what happens to your whole body when your sugar gets too high. The blood can't get out to where it is needed. This lack of blood is just plain bad everywhere, but some parts of your body are affected earlier than others. Your brain, tendons and liver are especially vulnerable.

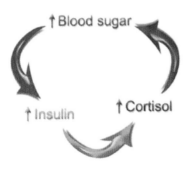

Along with not feeling well, we have to work hard when our sugar moves out of range. Hormones like cortisol and insulin are used to push our sugar up or down. They both work to control our blood sugar, but when we need a lot of them, they make us stressed and overweight. This is because they don't fine-tune our sugar levels, but rather make them bounce above and below the range.

Insulin is a storage hormone. The more of it you make, the more apt you are to store calories around your belly. Cortisol is a stress hormone. The more of it you make, the more apt you are to feel stressed, tired and anxious. The more your blood sugar swings up, the more it drops down. The more it drops down, the more cravings you will get for sugar.

If we can keep it in this tight range of 70-100 we can have:
• Great energy levels
• Reduction in belly fat
• Lower risk of chronic diseases
• Less cravings for sweets

Okay, so how do you do this? For most, the most powerful initial step is a high protein breakfast.

This works best when you have a reasonable amount of food for breakfast that yields a high amount of protein. If you have four pastries, you may end up with 20 grams of protein but at the cost of too many calories.

The foods that give you the most protein per calorie include seafood, poultry, lean meat, cottage cheese, nonfat unsweetened Greek yogurt, eggs, and unsweetened protein powders.

Protein for breakfast? Traditional Japanese commonly started their days with fish, vegetables and some rice. That may not sound good to you, but if you tried to sell them on pancakes, butter, syrup and juice for breakfast, they would be just as shocked. Somewhere along the way, we got the bad idea that the best way to start the day is with dessert or nothing at all.

The magic amount of protein is 30 grams. If you get it, your blood sugar will stay much steadier for the whole day.

Here are some easy options:
• 1.25 cups of unsweetened nonfat Greek yogurt = 30 grams
• 1.5 serving of VegaPro™ vegetable protein powder = 36 grams
• 1 egg, plus 1 cup liquid egg white = 32 grams
• 3.5 ounces of chicken breast = 30 grams
• 4 ounces of salmon = 30 grams

If you have some combination of fatigue, food cravings, insomnia, anxiety, headaches, muscle pain and poor short-term memory, think about your blood sugar levels.

If you'd like to get more lean and focused, think about your blood sugar levels.

Would you like to plan for great health and smooth aging? Have our doctors evaluate your insulin, cortisol and blood sugar. If anything is not ideal, it can be soon!

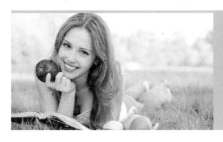

Fructose Vindicated for Obesity Epidemic?

By Dr. Alan Christianson

A recent meta-analysis published in the *Annals of Internal Medicine* looked at more than 40 fructose studies and concluded this sugar may not be a metabolic villain after all.

In some of these studies, participants either consumed fructose or another sugar. Regardless of what sugar they ate, their weight gain was about equivalent. In other words, the fructose did not create any additional gain.

In the other studies, researchers divided people into a regular group (where they ate their normal diet) or a fructose group (where they ate their normal diet plus fructose). The group that added fructose gained more weight.

Based on these studies, researchers concluded fructose was not any more fattening than other sugars. However, they admitted the studies they examined had problems: they were too small, for instance, or were otherwise poor quality.

Another problem is that these studies only used fructose. In reality, you consume fructose combined with glucose, such as table sugar or high fructose corn syrup.

Fructose and glucose do different things in your body. Glucose triggers insulin release. On the other hand, fructose heads to your liver, where it's poorly metabolized and eventually gets repackaged as triglycerides.

Eating too much of either sugar can trigger weight gain, a weakened immune system, and numerous other problems.

There's a huge difference between sugars in whole and processed foods. Whole foods like fruit are what nature intended you to eat, and come packed with fiber and nutrients. When you eat, say, an apple, you don't usually have fructose's problems.

But most sugar today comes in packaged foods via high fructose corn syrup. You want zero of this sugar, which creates all sorts of metabolic havoc and provides none of the nutrients whole foods provide.

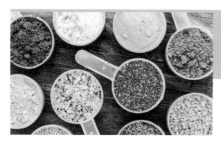

Alternatives to HCG

By Dr. Linda Khoshaba

Human Chorionic Gonadotropin, known as hCG, is a natural hormone produced during pregnancy. In the last few years, hCG has been used as a popular weight loss agent. This hormone is believed to prevent the body from going into starvation mode while a low calorie diet is maintained. The average number of calories on this diet varies from 500 to 1000 per day, mostly consisting of vegetable and protein sources. The hormone is administered daily through either oral drops or injections. A person can expect to lose anywhere from 1 to 2 pounds per day, which sounds like a fast and easy way for someone to lose the weight they have always dreamed of!

Despite all the great ideas of the hCG diet, there is no scientific evidence that it is effective and safe for weight loss and reducing hunger. There may be dangers associated with this diet, such as the development of a condition known as deep vein thrombosis, along with increases in certain types of cancers. There are alternatives to this diet that are safe, effective and help you keep the weight off long-term, so take a second to think twice about it!

Alternative #1

You keep hearing it over and over again, but nothing is better than diet and exercise. Slow and steady exercise and healthy eating are the best and safest proven methods to help sustain permanent weight loss. But the word diet itself can have endless meanings. The best diet consists of eating foods that are high in nutritious vitamins and minerals that will help your body stay healthy. Before you go on a healthy food shopping spree, it may be beneficial to have your food allergies tested so that you know what diet is best for your body. A food allergy test can be performed at a doctor's office, where you can get tested for numerous types of foods ranging from dairy, meat, fruits, vegetables, and grains. This type of allergy test looks for immune reactions to antigens in foods. Although you may think that you don't have food allergies because you don't have an anaphylactic reaction to certain foods, you still may have an internal immune reaction that has more subtle symptoms. Food allergies can create underlying inflammation in the intestinal tract and can lead to a condition known as Leaky Gut. This is where the gastrointestinal tract does not absorb vitamins and minerals from food properly, which can affect how your body breaks down sugar and uses it for energy. This can be an obstacle for you to lose weight.

Once you get your food allergy results, then it would be a good time to go shopping and familiarize yourself with the labels and items in the grocery store and avoid the foods that you may be reacting to. In the meantime, focus on getting your intestines healthy again so you can be on track with your overall health and lose weight the right way!

Alternative #2

Protein powders and shakes may be a safer and better alternative than the hCG diet. You may think that only athletes or body builders use these products to help them build muscle and get in shape, but they can be a safe and easy alternative for many people who are trying to get into better shape. Before you start this type of meal replacement, check with your doctor to make sure you are a candidate for this. A good protein powder consists of hypoallergenic ingredients that are dairy-free, gluten-free, and soy-free; usually rice and/or pea protein. The amount of protein can vary from 20-25 grams of protein per serving, and often provides other key ingredients such as a multivitamin, probiotics, and detox factors that help support your liver. So not only are you getting a great source of nutrition, you are losing weight in the process. The way that a protein powder diet usually works is that a person can have a protein shake for breakfast and/or lunch, and then usually a "lean and green" meal for dinner. The "lean and green" part of this diet allows you to eat a nutritious meal that is free of sugars and allergens and is basically any type of protein source paired with fresh vegetables made to your style. Not only are you getting the benefits of reducing inflammation in your body, your blood sugars will be more stable, you will detox and lose weight. And the best part is that it's easy!

HCG Alternatives

Protein powders and shakes may be a safer and better alternative than the hCG diet.

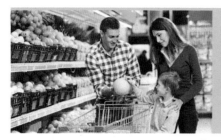

Navigating the Grocery Store and Planning a Nutritious Dinner

By Dr. Alan Christianson

We've all been in this situation before. You're on your way home from work, school, or some other daytime commitment, and suddenly you realize... you forgot to plan dinner! In the hustle and bustle of our daily lives, it seems nearly impossible to make healthy food choices, but planning a nutritious meal is easier than you think!

There seems to be a growing misconception in our new eco-conscious culture that, in order to maintain a healthy diet, you must revert back to the lifestyle of a nineteenth century subsistence farmer. However, for the vast majority of us, that is simply not a practical solution. The good news is, a nutritious dinner can still be found within the four walls of your neighborhood supermarket. You just have to know where to look!

Navigating a grocery store nowadays can be a little overwhelming, especially when you're hunting for a healthy option. You just don't have time to read the labels for the tens of thousands of products. One easy trick when shopping for a nutritious meal: start at the perimeter.

Around the perimeter of the grocery store is typically where you find the fresh, unprocessed staples of a healthy dinner. Lining the walls of the store, you've got the bakery, the deli, the produce section, and the dairy cooler, filled with simple, fresh options that pack a nutritious punch.

This is not to say you should completely ignore the entire middle section of the supermarket. There are good things to be found in the aisles as well. Just really keep a look out for what you're actually buying. While the colors, flavors, and textures may be different, a lot of processed foods on the shelves actually contain the same basic ingredients: wheat flour, corn flour, corn syrup, hydrogenated oils, salt, and enemy number one of our modern food system, MSG.

Yes, MSG is a preservative in many of the processed foods you buy at the grocery store. You just might not recognize it in the list of ingredients on the back of the box. It is sometimes written as monosodium glutamate, its full name, but it is also labeled as hydrolyzed soy extract, natural flavorings, natural additives, and other deceiving names.

So that is why it's usually best to begin planning your meal by walking the perimeter and selecting items that are fresh and unprocessed first. It's an easy way to add variety and essential nutrients to your diet.

So you know where to look, but what should you look for? What do you really want to serve on your plate for dinner? It's actually as easy as 1-2-3.
• Produce
• Protein
• Starch

Produce for Health

Produce is a key component of a healthy meal. In fact, it's so important that about half of your dinner should be produce. A good rule of thumb for measuring out your produce without actually having to measure anything: serve a portion equivalent to about two hands worth of produce for your meal. One of the biggest health benefits of a diet rich in produce is the antioxidants. Antioxidants help negate the harmful effects of the unpaired electrons, called free radicals, our body produces when generating energy. Look for colorful, nutrient-dense produce, such as carrots, sweet potatoes, broccoli, spinach, and yellow and red bell peppers. These are all great additions to a dinner and don't require a lot of prep time!

Protein is another important part of the meal. In the body, protein is an important part of every cell, so it makes sense that protein is essential in our diet. Going back to our rule of thumb again, an appropriate protein portion should be about the size of your palm. The best options for protein are the ones that are low in fat and less processed, things like salmon, white meat poultry, and shellfish. Red meat is not a bad thing for variety. Just try to cut out the fat, because that's where the toxins are concentrated. When it comes to choosing from these things, wild and organic are better choices for avoiding pesticides, antibiotics, and other contaminants. For all you vegetarians and vegans out there, try tempeh, tofu, hummus, and other meat alternatives to fill your protein needs. Eggs can be a good source of protein too. Milk, yogurt, and cheese don't really count as protein, as they provide more carbohydrate, sugar, and fat calories than they do protein calories. A variety of protein options await you in the butcher, deli, and organic sections of the grocery store. Don't be afraid to try something new!

Starch is the final piece of the puzzle. Now, starch has become the target of some nutritionists, like 'anti-carbohydrate' dietician Dr. Atkins, but the reality is that starch is an essential component of our diet. You just have to know how to incorporate it. The rule of thumb for starches is you want the portion to be about the size of your fist. Starches are the biggest source of fuel for your body. The key is to incorporate unprocessed, slow-burning carbohydrates that are high in fiber into your meal. Things like oatmeal, whole grain pasta, beans, brown rice, and quinoa are the perfect addition to your meal and add to the variety of your menu. Even at the end of the day, it is important to maintain your energy level by including an appropriate amount of starch in your dinner.

So, those are the 1-2-3's of a successful shopping experience for your next dinner. Start with the perimeter sections of the grocery store. Incorporate variety and color into your meal. Try to utilize the freshest ingredients. Follow the simple proportion rules. But, most of all, enjoy a great homemade meal!

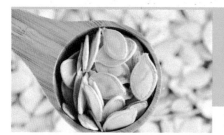

One of the Best Foods – Pumpkin Seeds

By Dr. Alan Christianson

One of the best foods you may be missing: Pumpkin Seeds
Pumpkin seeds are tasty and among the very highest source of some hard-to-get minerals, especially magnesium and zinc. They are also rich in copper, vitamin E and other antioxidants.

In addition to the nutrients, pumpkin seeds have unique phytosterols that may benefit cholesterol levels and prostate function.

How to use:
The most nutritional forms are the whole seed with the outer shell present

The membrane just inside of this is the source of many of the minerals. That is removed when the shell is taken off, but the shelled green seeds are still high in antioxidants and phytosterols.

Pumpkins are great foods, and these nutritional profiles are nearly interchangeable with squash seeds. Take a pumpkin or a squash, remove the seeds, and rinse. Take the rinsed seeds and shake in a bag with 1 tsp. powdered sea salt.

Where do you get powdered sea salt, you may ask? Take good sea salt and run it dry in your blender, 1-2 cups at a time for one minute. Ta Da!

Next spread the seeds on a baking sheet and bake in a 250 degree oven for 30 minutes. They're amazing!

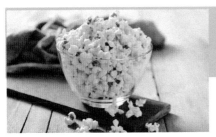

Crunchy, Salty and Healthy!

By Dr. Alan Christianson

Who likes salty, crunchy snacks?
Who doesn't!

Did you know that the densest known source of calories by weight is potato chips? Seriously, if you're trying to summit Everest, this is the best thing to pack. If you're trying to lose weight and be healthy, not such a good idea.

But fear not, here is a cool recipe for a crunchy, salty snack that is totally healthy and delicious. We start with popcorn. You don't want microwave popcorn due to perfluorooctanoic acid. Trust me – a bad thing.

Of course you don't want packaged or movie popcorn – way too much bad fat and salt. Air popped is reasonable, but not tasty unless you pour on tons of butter and salt.

Get some good quality organic popcorn and an old fashioned Whirley Pop™. These are available in kitchen supply stores or online, and they work great.

Next, get some Lite-Salt™ and xylitol. Lite-Salt™ is potassium and sodium. Xylitol is a healthy sugar substitute. Separately blend about a cup of each in your blender with no liquid for about a minute. They will form a fine powder. Store each in separate containers.

Take 1 – 2 tsp. macadamia nut oil or coconut oil and use to place a thin coat on the bottom of the popper. Add 1/2 cup popcorn and 2 tsp. Lite-Salt™.

Heat on a high flame and turn the stirring paddle for 2 minutes. Once popping starts, quickly pour in 1/2 cup of xylitol and continue stirring until popping stops.

Ta-Da! You've got 'kettle corn' but without excess fat, salt or sugar. Try it! It might become a new addiction.

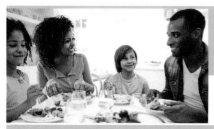

Sample Healthy Recipes

By Dr. Alan Christianson

Breakfast

BREAKFAST SHAKE

Blend all ingredients in high-powered blender with ½ cup each ice and water (add more water if you prefer your shakes thinner)

Ingredients

1 serving sugar free, vegetable based protein powder

1/2 cup frozen berries

1/2 cup unsweetened coconut milk beverage

1 Tbs. flaxseed

½ cup frozen spinach

Breakfast Shake Substitution options:

Instead of coconut, use unsweetened flax or almond milk.
Chia, hemp, salvia, or pumpkin seeds instead of flaxseed.
Kale, collards or other greens can replace spinach.

BREAKFAST PARFAIT

When you are in a rush but want something solid, parfaits are a perfect fit.

Yield: 4 servings as main dish	Prep time: 3 minutes	Cook time: n/a

Ingredients

2 cups nonfat unsweetened coconut yogurt

2 servings of vanilla flavored vegetable-based protein powder

½ cup oat bran

½ cup flaxseed

1 cup diced banana (to prevent insulin reactions use under-ripe bananas with green on the skin)

1/8 tsp. almond extract

Liquid stevia or powdered xylitol to taste

Instructions

Mix all dry ingredients in 1 quart mixing bowl. Stir in almond extract. Add in stevia or xylitol to optimal taste.

Vegan modifications: Serve with coconut yogurt

Make a batch, throw it in the refrigerator and you have a week's worth of breakfast cooked. Besides, soups always taste even better after they have had some time to let flavors mingle. They work great along with or instead of a smoothie on the busy days.

This is one of our favorite and easiest breakfasts. Any leftover vegetables can be added in as optional ingredients. You can also add quinoa or brown rice for a great complete meal later in the day.

Yield: 4 servings as main dish	Prep time: 3 minutes	Cook time: 2 minutes

Ingredients

2 medium-sized ripe avocados, pitted and peeled	2 chicken breasts, cooked and diced (precooked white meat can be used)
1 quart organic chicken or vegetable broth	½ tsp. dried turmeric
	½ tsp. dried ginger

Instructions

Blend avocados, broth and turmeric until smooth. Pour into 2 quart saucepan Add chicken. Gently heat until warm.

CHOCOLATE PUDDING

This is an amazing dish that even the fussiest of eaters will love. Please note this is one you make the night before and let refrigerate overnight.

Yield: 4 servings as main dish	Prep time: 3 minutes	Cook time: n/a

Ingredients

2 cups unsweetened coconut milk	½ cup chia seeds
1 banana, unripe with some green skin	½ cup sunflower seeds
	1 tsp. vanilla extract
¼ cup of cocoa powder (can use carob powder for those who are caffeine sensitive)	Liquid stevia or lo han (monk fruit) powder to taste
1 serving vanilla flavor vegetable-based protein powder	

Instructions

Mix all liquid ingredients in 1 quart mixing bowl. Dice the banana, stir in remaining ingredients. Add in stevia or monk fruit to optimal taste. Cover and place in refrigerator overnight, serve chilled.

BREAKFAST CHILI

Chili for breakfast? Try it and see how much your metabolism skyrockets! With spices, resistant fiber, veggies and quality protein, this will power your day like no other. This is my favorite breakfast. Typically I'll make up a large batch on Sunday evening and be set on breakfast for the coming week. Each morning requires just a minute to warm it up.

Yield: 4 servings as main dish	Prep time: 3 minutes	Cook time: 10 minutes

Ingredients

1 pound 95% lean or leaner ground beef or turkey	1 cup black beans, cooked and rinsed (canned are fine)
1-2 Tbs. macadamia oil or grape seed oil	2 cups arugula leaves or other greens
1 cup of your favorite mild salsa (look for lower salt and sugar free – salsa verde makes an exotic taste)	Optional ingredients: just about any vegetables. Great ones include onions, mushrooms, cabbage, celery or green chilies.
1-3 Tbs. chili powder	

Instructions

Brown meat in a 2 quart saucepan in the oil. Add salsa, chili powder, beans and spinach. Gently heat until arugula leaves are wilted. **Optional garnishes:** diced onion, cilantro, parsley, lime

LOWER CARB MUESLI

Maximilian Bircher-Benner was a Swiss physician who developed Muesli around the turn of the last century as a breakfast to use for patients in his hospital. It was inspired from a mixture he and his wife used while hiking in the Swiss Alps. Oats are used in this low carb recipe. In a raw state, they are high enough in resistant starch to not cause significant insulin production.

Yield: 4 servings as main dish	Prep time: 3 minutes	Cook time: n/a

Ingredients

1 cup organic old fashioned oats	½ cup ground flaxseed
1 cup shredded, unsweetened coconut flakes	½ cup freeze dried unsweetened blueberries
1 serving vanilla flavored vegetable based protein powder	1 tsp. vanilla extract
½ cup oat bran	liquid stevia to taste

Instructions

Mix all dry ingredients in 1 quart mixing bowl. Stir in vanilla. Add in stevia to optimal taste. **Optional garnishes:** can serve with ½ cup unsweetened coconut beverage.

LUNCH SALAD

Ingredients

4 cups Romaine, red leaf, green leaf lettuce	6 cherry tomatoes
	1 Tbs. olive oil
½ cup black beans	2 Tbs. red wine vinegar
3 ounces canned salmon	½ tsp. Spike® seasoning

Instructions

Rinse beans and salmon. Mix all ingredients together. Keep chilled until serving. Salad Substitution options: You can use any other greens instead of lettuce. Try any other type of beans. Chickpeas and navy beans are great options. Chicken, shrimp, tempeh or other protein can be used in place of the salmon. You can use any other vinegar with the exception of flavored or balsamic vinegar. (If you are not sure if vinegar is flavored just check the label. If total carbs are over 1 gram per serving, it is flavored.) Other oils can be used instead of olive oil. Other seasoning blends can replace Spike®. (If you are not familiar with it, try Spike®.)

SALMON WALDORF SALAD

Waldorf salads come in all types but the original base includes apples, walnuts and celery. This version is quick to prepare and makes a complete meal – perfect for lunch. This recipe will make enough for you and a spouse or child. You can also keep it all for yourself and eat ½ for lunch the following day. If you do plan to save some, be sure to wait until you are ready to eat it to add the dressing.

Yield: 2 servings as main dish	Prep time: 10 minutes	Cook time: n/a

Ingredients

6 cups washed and torn lettuce (try any blend of escarole, endive or romaine)	1 Granny Smith apple, diced
	6 walnut halves
	2 ribs of celery, diced
6 ounces canned wild salmon packed in water	½ cup garbanzo beans, rinsed

Dressing

Soy-Free Veganaise® brand egg-free mayonnaise

Instructions

Mix all ingredients in 2 quart mixing bowl.
Stir in dressing prior to serving.

SOUTHWEST CHIPOTLE SALAD

Chipotle is a seasoning made from smoked jalapeno peppers, which have a totally unique smoky flavor. Do not despair if you are not a fan of spicy foods. Small amounts of chipotle give more flavor than heat. This salad works great to make a few days' worth in advance and add the dressing before serving.

Yield: 4 servings as main dish	Prep time: 15 minutes	Cook time: n/a

Ingredients

8 cups washed and torn greens (try any blend of romaine spinach or shredded cabbage)

2 diced chicken breasts (can also use pre-cooked chicken)

½ cup finely sliced red onion

2 cups broccoli florets

1 cup cherry tomatoes (these work great in pre-made salads and keep it from getting soggy)

2 cups black beans, rinsed

Dressing

½ cup non-fat unsweetened coconut yogurt

1 ripe avocado, peeled and seeded

1/3 cup lemon juice

1 clove garlic

¼ - ½ tsp ground chipotle or few shakes of Tabasco® brand Chipotle flavored hot sauce

Instructions

Mix all ingredients in 2 quart mixing bowl. Stir in dressing prior to serving.

LENTIL PATE

Traditional French Pate is made from minced liver and seasonings and is served on toast. This is a self-contained meal with a similar flavor, but with tons of fiber, good quality protein and lots of antioxidants. You can whip up a couple of batches of these in no time and have a portable and tasty lunch ready to go.

Yield: 12 Pates as main dish 2-3 per serving	Prep time: 10 mins	Cook time: 30 mins

Ingredients

1 cup green lentils, cooked or canned

6 ounces of diced chicken breast

2 cups sliced button mushrooms

1 red bell pepper, diced

1 small red onion, diced

2 cloves garlic minced

½ tsp. sea salt

½ tsp. pepper

½ tsp. chili powder

½ tsp. turmeric

Macadamia or grape seed oil

Instructions

Preheat oven to 350 degrees Fahrenheit. Sauté mushrooms, red pepper and onion in sauté pan with 1-2 tsp. of oil. Add seasonings when vegetables soften. Mix all ingredients in 2 quart mixing bowl. Spoon into lightly oiled muffin tins, filling nearly to the top. Bake for 20-25 minutes or until firm.

SPINACH BEAN SOUP WITH PRAWNS

Here is another great lunch dish that can be made in the morning or in advance. Bring a batch for your co-workers; they will be amazed at your culinary skills. You don't have to tell them that it only took 10 minutes. Note that this recipe uses canned coconut milk for cooking. This is not the same as the coconut beverage in soft packs.

Yield: 4 servings	Prep time: 10 minutes	Cook time: 10 minutes

Ingredients

1 can (1 ½ cups) coconut milk	1 clove garlic, minced
1 can black beans	½ tsp. sea salt
6 cups washed spinach leaves	½ tsp. pepper
½ cup raw cashews, chopped	1 tsp. chili powder
1 pound prawns, cooked and tails removed	1 pinch cayenne pepper
	Macadamia or grape seed oil
1 small red onion, diced	

Instructions

Sauté onion in 2-quart saucepan with 1-2 tsp. of oil. When onions start to soften, add prawns and cook for 1 minute. Add all remaining ingredients and stir in spinach until wilted. Simmer 10 minutes.

Dinner

DINNER STIR-FRY

Ingredients

1 cup brown rice	½ cup onions
3 ounces chicken breast	1 tsp. soy sauce
1 cup broccoli	2 tsp. toasted sesame oil
½ cup mushrooms	1 clove garlic, chopped

Instructions

Rice and chicken breast can be cooked in advance or purchased pre-cooked. Heat half of the oil in saucepan or wok. Heat garlic and onions for 1 minute. Add vegetables and cook until slightly soft. Add chicken, rice, soy sauce and remainder of sesame oil until all ingredients are mixed and warm.

Stir Fry Substitution options
Any other unlimited vegetables can be used. Try lean beef, pork or tempeh instead of chicken. Other oils can replace toasted sesame seed oil (macadamia oil works well in stir-frys). Other seasonings in place of soy sauce, such as Ume plum vinegar (although soy is generally avoided, natural soy sauce is fermented and fine in normal quantities).

GROUND TURKEY CASSEROLE

If your evenings are really tight, consider prepping this in the morning and putting it in to bake when you get home. This one has a handwritten 'A+' in our family cookbook. Cook the quinoa ahead of time or buy it pre-cooked.

Yield: 4 servings	Prep time: 10 minutes	Cook time: 30 minutes

Ingredients

1 can navy beans (1 ½ cups)	1 cup vegetable broth or Better than Bouillon
½ pounds ground turkey, lean	
1 cup coconut beverage	½ tsp. sea salt
1 cup sweet onion, diced	½ tsp. pepper
1 ½ cups sliced carrots or pre-shredded	1 tsp. turmeric powder
	1 tsp. coriander powder
1 ½ cups of asparagus cut into 1-inch pieces	2 cups quinoa, cooked
	Macadamia or grape seed oil
2 cups green cabbage, shredded	

Instructions

Preheat oven to 350 degrees Fahrenheit. Sauté ground turkey in skillet with 1-2 tsp. of oil. In a blender, combine navy beans, ½ the coconut milk, spices, blend until smooth. Mix cooked turkey, contents of blender and all ingredients in a large casserole dish. Bake uncovered for 25-30 minutes

Serve with: This can be a stand-alone dish or can go with a mixed green salad.

SEASONED RICE AND VEGGIES

Even if you are not a vegetarian or vegan, it is fine to have the occasional vegetarian dinner. Make sure it is high in fiber and has some healthy carbohydrates, and stick with a single serving.

Yield: 4 servings as main dish	Prep time: 10 minutes	Cook time: 55 minutes

Ingredients

1 cup brown rice, dry	½ cup zucchini, sliced
2 cups vegetable broth	½ cup red pepper, sliced
1 Tbs. miso	1 tsp. grated ginger
2 tsp. toasted sesame oil	1/3 cup pine nuts
1 cup mushrooms, quartered	
½ cup white onion, diced	

Optional garnish: ¼ cup diced cilantro

Instructions

Rinse rice. Add rice and broth to 2-quart sauce pan. Cover and simmer gently for 55 minutes. Sautee all remaining ingredients in sauce pan with toasted sesame oil. Fold vegetables into rice and serve.

CURRIED GARBANZO STEW

Curry is a blend of spices, usually built around turmeric. There is a compound found in turmeric called curcumin that can do more for your health than almost anything. It improves blood sugar control, lowers inflammation and helps the immune system. In fact, extracts of curcumin work as well for pain and inflammation as medications like ibuprofen, and without the side effects.

Yield: 4 servings as main dish	Prep time: 5 minutes	Cook time: 10 minutes

Ingredients

1 ½ cups brown basmati rice, cooked	1 Tbs. lemon juice
14 ounces canned garbanzo beans, rinsed	2 tsp. macadamia or grape seed oil
	1 cup white onion, diced
1 cup pureed tomatoes	2 tsp. cumin seeds
2 cups cabbage, chopped	1 tsp. grated ginger
½ jalapeno pepper, seeded and minced (wash your hands after handling)	1 Tbs. grated ginger
	½ tsp. sea salt

Optional garnish: ½ cup diced cilantro

Instructions

Sauté mustard and cumin seeds in oil until they pop. Add cabbage, onion, ginger and jalapeno; cook until all have softened. Add tomatoes, turmeric and garbanzo beans. Simmer for 5-10 minutes. Serve over rice.

SPICY PEANUT "NOODLES"

Ingredients

1 lb. mung bean sprouts	1 inch piece fresh ginger, peeled and grated
3 stalks celery, sliced	
2 cups mushrooms, sliced	Red pepper flakes, to taste
1 bunch green onions	2 Tbs. natural peanut butter
1 Tbs. toasted sesame oil	

Instructions

Heat oil in a large skillet. Add celery, green onions and mushrooms. Sautee until softened and liquids released. Add in mung bean sprouts, ginger, and pepper flakes to taste. Cover and steam sprouts, stirring occasionally. When sprouts have cooked down, stir in peanut butter until dissolved.

AFTER SUMMER RATATOUILLE

Ingredients

1 Tbs. olive oil	1-2 yellow squash, diced
2 garlic cloves, peeled and minced	1 eggplant, diced
1 sweet onion, diced	1 red bell pepper, diced
1 cup water	8 oz mushrooms, quartered
1 cup cherry tomatoes, halved	1 Tbs. ground thyme
1 zucchini, diced	1 cup organic marinara sauce
	1/4 cup fresh basil, finely chopped

Instructions

In a large pot, heat the olive oil, garlic and onion over medium heat for about 2 minutes. Add cherry tomatoes and cook until they start breaking down. Add water and season with salt and pepper. Add remaining vegetables and continue to cook for about 10 minutes until vegetables are tender, but still a bit firm. Stir in marinara sauce and continue cooking until heated through, about 3-4 minutes. Season to taste with black pepper and stir in fresh basil.

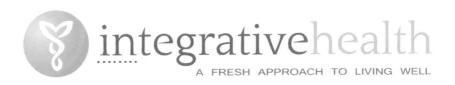

integrative health
A FRESH APPROACH TO LIVING WELL

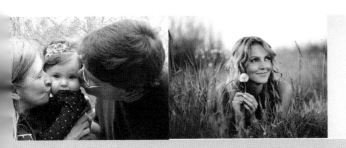
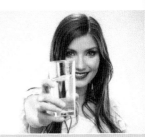

Chapter 6: Beauty & Detox

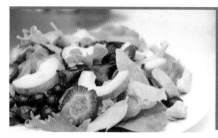

Skin Food: 5 Foods for a Radiant Glow from the Inside Out

By Dr. Adrienne Stewart

Radiant skin starts from the inside out. The skin needs proper nutrition to repair damage caused by the sun and pollution, to maintain its moisture and elasticity, and to keep fine lines and wrinkles at bay. Some basics for radiant skin include eating a whole foods diet, getting enough sleep, exercise, and proper skin care. But, to really power up your lifestyle for healthy, glowing skin, try adding these four things into your diet.

Avocado

Avocado is a power-packed skin food. As a good source of omega-3 and omega-6, it provides the skin with the nutrients it needs to maintain moisture and elasticity. These essential fatty acids also help reduce inflammation, which can minimize puffiness around the eyes. These healthy fats also unlock the antioxidant properties in other vegetables when eaten in combination. Research shows that adding avocado to a salad of spinach, tomatoes, romaine, and carrots will increase the absorption of carotenoids and lycopene by more than 200%. But even on their own, avocados are a rich source of unique antioxidants that help support the body in many ways. In addition to essential fatty acids and antioxidants, avocados are also rich in fiber, vitamin K, vitamin C, and the B vitamins. The most nutrient-dense part of the avocado is in the dark green flesh right under the skin. So, the best way to peel one is with your fingers. Try adding avocado to salads, thicken up soups with avocado puree, add it to smoothies for a creamy texture, or make a veggie-packed guacamole.

Blueberries

Blueberries are antioxidant-packed, helping your skin recover from environmental damage caused by free radicals. Blueberries have a wide variety of antioxidants and phytonutrients with impressive names like: anthocyanins, hydroxycinnamic acids, hydroxybenzoic acids, and flavonols. These nutrients help the body repair damage caused by overexposure to sun, pollution, toxins, and other environmental stressors that rob our skin of its radiance. While many fruits and vegetables contain antioxidants, blueberries shine because they have such a wide variety of nutrients, because they do not lose potency when frozen, and because they do not negatively affect blood sugar, despite being sweet. This makes them not only nutritious, but convenient for modern lifestyles. To add more blueberries to your diet, try adding them to oatmeal, cereal, or pancakes in the morning, eat them as a midday snack, top salads, yogurts, or even blend them into a smoothie.

Papaya
Papaya provides one of the highest sources of vitamin C, with more than 300% of your daily allowance in a single fruit. Vitamin C is critical for radiant skin because of its ability to repair collagen, which protects you from premature aging and sun damage. Papaya also contains vitamin E, another critical skin nutrient. The antioxidant properties of vitamin E help protect your cells from the damage caused by free radicals, and have cancer-fighting properties. In addition to its vitamin content, papaya is full of antioxidants that do wonders for your skin. To get the most antioxidant benefits, it's best to eat papayas when they are completely ripe. They should have a red to orange tinge on their skin and be moderately soft to touch. Add papaya to your diet by including it in salads, smoothies, desserts, or eating it fresh as a snack. People with a severe latex allergy should avoid eating papayas, along with avocados, bananas, chestnuts, and kiwi.

Water
Water is essential for radiant skin because of its ability to both hydrate the skin and help flush out toxins in your system that may cause breakouts. If you increase your intake of any kind of fruit or vegetable, such as avocados, blueberries, or papayas, it is important to also increase your water intake. Fruits and vegetables have a high fiber content that can absorb water in your body. This can dry out your skin and break collagen strands, which increase signs of aging. Water also helps the detox pathways in the body get rid of unwanted waste and toxins that can cause breakouts. Try drinking at least half your body weight in ounces per day, in addition to any other beverages you are drinking.

Water

Water is essential for radiant skin because of its ability to both hydrate the skin and help flush out toxins in your system that may cause breakouts.

Flaxseed
Flaxseed is excellent if you experience hormonal outbreaks. Flaxseed is rich in a phytonutrient called lignans. Lignans have antioxidant properties, fiber-like benefits, and can even act as safe phytoestrogens in the body. Flaxseed also is high in essential fatty acids, which help with inflammation. Among their myriad health benefits, they also help improve inflammation due to acne by

helping to regulate hormones and blood sugar levels. Flaxseed can be added to salads, muffins, soups, or even smoothies. It is best to grind up a small batch as you use it to keep it as fresh as possible.

Try out this smoothie recipe for the healthy glow of radiant skin:
Radiant Skin Smoothie
- 1 avocado
- 1 cup cubed papaya (can be frozen)
- 1 cup frozen blueberries
- 10 oz water
- 2 tsp. ground flaxseed

Blend all ingredients together and enjoy!

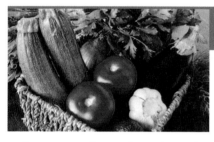

Avoiding Toxins

By Dr. Adrienne Stewart

We are exposed to toxins every day that disrupt the body's natural processes, from household cleaners to beauty products. Over time, these toxins can accumulate in our bodies. Some people retain more toxins than others due to stress, specific nutrient deficiencies, high-sugar and low-protein diets, increased exposures, difficulty excreting waste, and genetic differences.

While we cannot completely eliminate our exposure to toxins, it is possible to make a significant impact by limiting daily exposure. Many of these toxins disrupt immune function, hormone balance, and neurological function. With some simple changes, you can improve your, and your family's, health.

Avoiding Toxins in Food

Some foods expose you to toxins like pesticides and other chemicals. It is important to buy organic whole foods whenever possible. The Environmental Working Group provides two lists to help you buy produce. The *Clean 15* ™ is a list of produce you can eat liberally because they contain the least amount of pesticides. The *Dirty Dozen Plus* ™ lists the produce that contains the most pesticides; you'll want to buy the organic version of these items.

One of the best ways to help the body eliminate toxins is to increase the amount of clean water in the diet. Remember, ***the solution for pollution is dilution.*** It is important to use glass bottles and containers instead of plastics, and avoid the epoxy linings inside metal food cans because they may contain hormone-disrupting BPA.

For extra detoxification, avoid sugar, eat more broccoli and other members of the Brassica family, and avoid fish with high mercury content such as farmed or Atlantic salmon, shark, swordfish, tuna, or sea bass. In addition, choose foods high in lean protein like wild, grass-fed, grass-finished meat that is free of hormones or antibiotics. Pea and rice protein are also great proteins for shakes and smoothies.

EWG's Shoppers Guide to Pesticides in Produce

Dirty Dozen Plus ™	
Apples	Peaches
Celery	Potatoes
Cherry tomatoes	Spinach
Cucumbers	Strawberries
Grapes	Sweet bell peppers
Hot peppers	Kale/collard greens
Nectarines (imported)	Summer squash

Clean Fifteen ™	
Asparagus	Mangos
Avocados	Mushrooms
Cabbage	Onions
Cantaloupe	Papayas
Sweet Corn	Pineapples
Eggplant	Sweet peas – frozen
Grapefruit	Sweet potatoes
Kiwi	

Avoiding Toxins at Home

Your home is another area where you may be exposed to toxins, also called indoor air pollution. Indoor toxins include cigarette smoke, chemicals that get tracked in on the bottom of your shoes, and off-gas from vinyl shower curtains, construction materials, new furniture, carpets, and dry cleaning. To clean up the indoor air quality, try HEPA air purifiers, carbon air filters, indoor houseplants, taking off shoes, proper air duct cleaning, and environmentally friendly construction materials. For your yard, there are lots of natural alternatives and companies that focus on healthier herbicides and pesticides. Also consider your car exhaust, workplace, and what potential toxins you are exposed to and could possibly avoid on a day-to-day basis.

Avoiding Toxins in Personal Care Products:

Other hidden toxins are the chemicals used in cosmetics, cleaners, laundry soaps, air fresheners, and other household products. Pay special attention to your personal care products because they are applied directly to your skin.

Avoid products with fragrances, dyes, and parabens. Your local health food store will have natural cosmetics, shampoos, and lotions. You can also check the quality of your current cosmetics in the EWG's Skin Deep Database. In addition, health food stores have all-natural household products like laundry soap and multi-purpose cleaners.

Okay, now what?
Now that you have limited your daily exposure, you can take cleansing a step further, if needed. A common test we do here at Integrative Health is a heavy metal test. Other testing may include checking levels of BPA, phthalates, and parabens. These tests can help determine your body burden and the depth of cleansing needed.

Cleansing may include specific diet protocols, targeted supplementation with liver support, and therapies such as sauna therapy, constitutional hydrotherapy, colon hydrotherapy, or heavy metal chelation.

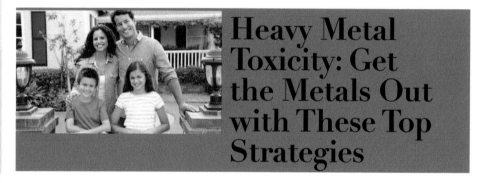

Heavy Metal Toxicity: Get the Metals Out with These Top Strategies

By Dr. Alan Christianson

A healthy diet and lifestyle are the most effective means to reduce your risk for diseases like cancer, diabetes, and heart disease, as well as Parkinson's and Alzheimer's diseases.

This includes plenty of organic fruits and vegetables, nuts and seeds, and quality protein like grass-fed beef and wild salmon. You also want to reduce or eliminate processed foods, sugar, and alcohol (other than red wine, which can be beneficial in moderation).

I also want you to exercise regularly. You needn't spend hours on an elliptical machine or spin classes to get exercise's benefits. Burst training gives you a full body workout in just minutes a day, and it becomes even more effective when you combine it with weight resistance.

Once you've covered those bases, the best thing you can do to reduce your disease risk involves eliminating heavy metal intake.

Heavy metal toxicity contributes to numerous diseases, and anyone living in the modern world is at risk. A study in the journal *Alternative Therapies in Health & Medicine* found that mercury and other toxic metals increase your risk for vascular disease, high blood pressure, and heart disease.

A 2007 and 2011 priority list on hazardous materials from the Center for Disease Control and Prevention (CDC) found the top hazardous substances included arsenic, lead, mercury, vinyl chloride, polychlorinated biphenyls, benzene, and cadmium.

You might know these metals are dangerous, but not know why. I want to briefly discuss how the top three metals can create serious health problems. Then I'll provide tips to reduce your risk for exposure and toxicity.

Arsenic

Tap water is a prevalent source of this toxic metal. In 2000, the National Resources Defense Counsel (NRDC) analyzed data compiled by the U.S. Environmental Protection Agency (EPA) on arsenic in drinking water in 25 states.

Arsenic

Tap water is a prevalent source of this toxic metal.

The results weren't good. Even the most conservative estimates showed more than 34 million Americans drink tap water supplied by systems containing arsenic levels that posed unacceptable cancer risks. Additionally, 56 million people in those 25 states were drinking water with arsenic at unsafe levels.

I want you to drink half your weight in water ounces every day, but always stick with purified water to avoid arsenic and other nasty metals sometimes prevalent in tap water.

Seafood can also be high in arsenic. I want you to eat seafood for all its health benefits, but choose the right kinds to reduce arsenic intake. High arsenic seafood sources include shellfish like shrimp, lobster, and scallops.

You're not off the hook (no pun intended) if you're a vegetarian. A study in the journal *Food and Chemical Toxicology* found hijiki seaweed has very high levels of inorganic arsenic.

So, why should you avoid these sources of arsenic? For one, arsenic in drinking water can cause skin, lung, bladder, and kidney cancers. Arsenic can also cause other skin changes such as thickening and pigmentation. A study in the *Journal of Exposure Science & Environmental Epidemiology* found increased risk of these cancers and skin changes in people drinking even small amounts (50 µg/litre, or even lower) of drinking water.

Lead

Agencies such as the CDC, ATSDR and the EPA all agree there is no safe level of lead. Even the tiniest amount can wreak havoc on your body.

Lead

According to an article in the journal *Circulation*, lead is the "silent killer." Agencies such as the CDC, the Agency for Toxic Substances and Disease Registry (ATSDR), and the Environmental Protection Agency (EPA) all agree there is no safe level of lead. In other words, even the tiniest amount can wreak havoc on your body.

That's because lead blocks your antioxidant enzymes, which can cause autoimmune diseases, unregulated inflammation, and increased levels of free radicals in tissue.

A systematic review of numerous lead studies in the journal *Environmental Health Perspectives* concluded that lead exposure could increase your risk for heart disease, and a disturbing study in the *Journal of Occupational and Environmental Medicine* linked lead with increased brain cancer risk.

So how do you know if you have lead toxicity? Early symptoms include:

- muscle weakness
- fatigue and lethargy
- attention deficit/ irritability
- muscle pain
- joint pain/arthritis
- appetite changes
- a metallic taste in your mouth

You should also become aware of later symptoms of lead toxicity, which include:

- headache
- insomnia
- irritability
- impaired libido
- weight gain of at least 10 pounds without any known cause
- nerve pain in arms and legs
- abdominal pain/cramping
- nausea/vomiting
- personality changes
- short-term memory loss
- depression

Pregnant and nursing moms – lead mobilization during pregnancy is hazardous to the fetus because this metal passes freely across the placenta. In fact, blood lead levels in the mother and fetus are usually identical.

Elderly people with osteoporosis – a study in the journal *Environmental Research* found a significant increase in lead concentration in postmenopausal women. Lead can also inhibit vitamin D activation and uptake of dietary calcium, increasing your risk for osteoporosis.

People with cataracts – a study in *The Journal of the American Medical Association (JAMA)*, showed 42% of cataracts are related to bone lead. The study concluded that reducing "lead exposure could help decrease the global burden of cataract."

Mercury

Mercury has deservedly earned a bad reputation. According to the World Health Organization (WHO), "Recent studies suggest that mercury may have no threshold below which some adverse effects do not occur." Just like with lead, even the tiniest amount of mercury can wreak havoc.

Mercury spares no system in your body, whether that means your nervous system, emotions, heart, kidneys, or hormones. Mercury can kill your sex drive and your immune system.

> "Recent studies suggest that mercury may have no threshold below which some adverse effects do not occur." – World Health Organization

The primary source of mercury is coal-fired power plants which, according to the EPA, emit more than 8,000 tons of mercury pollution per year.

Top sources of body mercury include vaccines, thermometers, fluorescent bulbs, skin creams, and dental amalgams. According to a study in JAMA, an amalgam contains 50% mercury.

Larger fish like tuna, swordfish, and shark also come loaded with mercury, which is especially prone to end up in your brain. Even small amounts can impair your ability to select words and process new information, and can worsen hand/eye coordination. In 1997, the EPA stated that at least eight percent of American women ages 16 to 49 carried dangerous levels of mercury in their bodies from seafood.

That's too bad, since eating fish provides excellent protein, good fats, and numerous nutrients like mercury-binding selenium. I want you to eat the right kind of fish in moderation. I recommend two meals with a total of up to 12 ounces of lower-mercury fish and shellfish every week. Low-mercury choices include shrimp, cod, canned wild salmon, Pollock, and catfish.

How much fish should I eat then?

We recommend two meals with a total of up to 12 ounces of fish in moderation.

Also keep in mind that albacore ("white") tuna has more mercury than canned light tuna, so limit albacore tuna to six ounces a week.

Speaking of food and mercury, I highly recommend you eliminate high fructose corn syrup (HFCS) from your diet. The average American eats a whopping 64 pounds of this sweetener every year, which can lead to diabetes and obesity.

Just as bad, a study in the journal *Environmental Health* found that half of foods tested with HFCS contain mercury, since many factories that produce HFCS use dated, low cost mercury-cell technologies.

Lifestyle measures
In addition to reducing or eliminating your exposure, I want you to give your body the proper nourishment to help effectively eliminate heavy metals and your risk for disease:

Clean up your diet. Eat sulfur-containing foods that help your liver detox, including broccoli, cabbage, onions, garlic, eggs, and non-denatured whey protein. I also recommend prebiotics, probiotics, and adequate fiber for optimal gut health. And choose a colorful array of organic vegetables, fruits, seeds, and nuts.

Get the right nutrients. Optimal amounts of nutrients from food can be challenging. That's why I suggest everyone take a high-quality multivitamin. Other nutrients that help detoxify metals include lipoic acid, N-acetyl cysteine (NAC), silymarin (milk thistle), and glutamine.

Clean up your environment. Install air filters in your home and cars, and water filters in your shower. Also use infrared saunas, which can help your body sweat out toxins.

Exercise. Speaking of sweating out toxins, nothing helps your body reduce heavy metal toxicity more than a good workout. I like burst training combined with weight resistance for efficient, effective exercise. While it may be fast, I promise you it's incredibly effective! But any kind of exercise that makes you sweat can also help you detoxify.

Reduce stress. Stress can damage your immune system and weaken your body's ability to eliminate heavy metals. Make time in your schedule every day to unwind, whether that means a hot bath, a massage, or taking a long walk with your dog.

Chelation. The word "chelate" comes from the Greek word chele, or claw, which makes sense, since chelation involves combining a metal ion with a chemical compound, forming a ring to eliminate the toxic metal. If you believe you suffer from symptoms related to heavy-metal toxicity, talk with a chelation specialist about potential measures you can take to reduce toxicity.

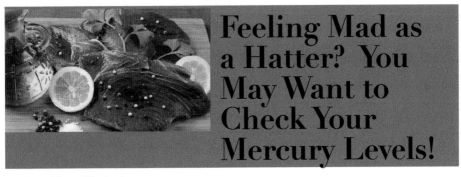

Feeling Mad as a Hatter? You May Want to Check Your Mercury Levels!

By Dr. Alan Christianson

In the 19th century, experienced hatters were famous for being erratic and delusional. Hatters spent the bulk of their workday leaning over hot cauldrons of mercuric nitrate, which was used to process felt into hats. Of course, this was done without today's requirements of ventilation or respirators, so the mercury they breathed in built up in their brains. Over time, they became rather odd.

Thank goodness we don't have to worry about such things today, right? Many obvious sources of mercury have been removed from our environment, but unfortunately, many still remain.

In fact, exposure to mercury is something you face every day. Even though we are only exposed to small amounts, our bodies cannot eliminate it, and over time it can build up. Who should be concerned about this?

Anyone who:
- Has more than 6 'silver' fillings
- Eats fish, especially tuna, more than 2 days a week
- Works with paints, cleaners, jewelry or agricultural chemicals

If you do get exposed to mercury, it often causes vague symptoms or contributes to other illnesses. Suspicious signs include:

- Erratic mood changes
- Hypothyroidism
- Memory loss
- Painful feet or hands
- Irritability
- Muscle weakness
- Episodes of confusion or disorientation
- Skin rashes

If so, mercury poisoning could be the source of your symptoms.

Today, our most common sources of exposure are:

- Dental amalgams
- Seafood
- High fructose corn syrup
- Medications

Check Your Fillings

Dental amalgams are silver colored fillings. They are made of 40-50% mercury.

Dental amalgams are silver colored fillings. They are made of 40-50% mercury. Amalgams gradually degrade and constantly leech mercury into your body. Amalgams are so toxic that the EPA has written elaborate procedures that dental labs must follow when disposing of any unused material.

Seafood contains a type of mercury that is especially prone to end up in our brains. Even small amounts have been shown to impair the ability to select words, to process new information, and worsen hand/eye coordination. The EPA was alarmed enough about this to issue a report to Congress in 1997, where they stated that at least 8% of American women ages 16-49 carried dangerous levels of mercury in their bodies from seafood.

Avoid seafood known to have the highest levels of mercury. These include mackerel, shark, swordfish and tilefish. Although tuna is not the highest source of mercury, it is a type of fish that many in the U.S. eat on a daily basis. The Environmental Working Group advises no more than 4 ounces of Tuna per week for most adults. Types of seafood lower in mercury include herring, pollock, wild salmon, sardines, shrimp and tilapia.

High fructose corn syrup (HFCS) is a sweetener widely used by food manufacturers. Many have argued that it is more dangerous than sugar. The increased use of HFCS over the last few decades has paralleled the rise in obesity over the same timeframe. It is now so common in our food that the average American eats ¼ - ½ cup of it every day!

A 2009 study showed that mercury was present in half of the foods containing HFCS. Many factories that produce HFCS still use dated but low cost mercury-cell technologies.

Many medications use mercury as a preservative. This is especially common in vaccines. The FDA has a list of over 130 prescription and over-the-counter medications which contain mercury. These include many eye drops, nasal sprays, skin creams and hemorrhoid ointments. Mercury is readily absorbed into the body from these sources.

Now that it is apparent we may be subject to daily mercury exposure, what can you do about it?

Even if you do not have symptoms of mercury toxicity, be aware of the sources and avoid what you can. This will lower your risk of harm and lower the global burden of mercury by supporting greener manufacturers.

Check Your Medications

Many medications use mercury as a preservative. This is especially common in vaccines. The FDA has a list of over 130 prescription and over-the-counter medications which contain mercury.

Further steps you can take include:
Replace any old or unstable dental amalgams with newer non-mercury alternatives.

Be aware of mercury in seafood. When you eat seafood, try to have foods like spinach and brown rice with it. This will cause you to absorb less mercury.

Avoid HFCS in your diet. Ask your doctor about mercury-free vaccines. They are available. Ask your pharmacist about mercury in eye drops, nasal and topical products. Mercury-free alternatives exist.

Because it is so hard for our bodies to eliminate mercury, reducing your intake alone is not always enough. If you may have had exposure, consider being tested. Some tests can be done at home without a doctor's order. These include hair tests and random urine tests. Hair tests are easy to do and non-invasive. Testing yourself is simple. Purchase a home kit from an online lab. Follow the directions on collecting a sample, and mail it back to the lab to be analyzed.

If the results show no mercury, most likely you do not have an excess. If they do show elevated mercury levels, you will need to be tested further by your doctor, as these home tests do not give you a perfect assessment of how much is actually in your body. Think of these online kits as yes or no tests. If they say yes, it is smart to do better testing.

There are two main ways your doctor will test for mercury

With and without provocation.

There are two main ways your doctor will test for mercury: with and without provocation. *With provocation* means a medicine that causes your body to eliminate mercury is given to you before urine is collected. This medicine pulls mercury from your tissues and fat cells, where it's been stored and allows the test to show how much mercury has built up in your body's organs over the years. *Unprovoked* tests are done without detox medicines. They show your last 1-3 days of exposure.

If mercury does show up, doctors trained in detoxification can guide you safely through a mercury detox process, so you will no longer feel as "mad as a hatter" and can enjoy life.

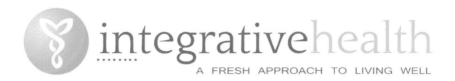
integrativehealth

A FRESH APPROACH TO LIVING WELL

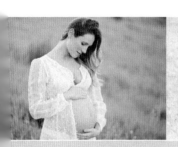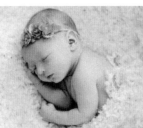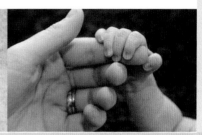

Chapter 7: Pregnancy & Pediatrics

Pre-Pregnancy Cleansing

By Dr. Adrienne Stewart

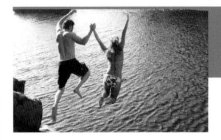

Preventative medicine has lifelong benefits. The earlier you invest in your health, the greater the returns you can expect throughout life. Imagine the benefits of beginning a healthy lifestyle as a young child or even before you were born. That is why preconception care can be very healing, not only for the mother and father, but also for the unborn child and future generations. One aspect of preconception care is cleansing the body. Some common chemicals we are exposed to everyday are toxins that disrupt the body's natural processes. Over time, these toxins can accumulate in our bodies. Some people retain more toxins than others due to stress, specific nutrient deficiencies, high sugar and low protein diets, increased exposures, difficulty excreting waste, and genetic differences. While we cannot completely eliminate our exposure to toxins, it is possible to make a significant impact by limiting daily exposure.

It is especially important for couples who want to conceive to be proactive about cleansing. Many of these toxins disrupt hormone balances, affecting fertility and delaying conception. Cleansing is safe before pregnancy, but not recommended once a woman becomes pregnant. With some simple changes, you can improve your health, and the health of your family.

In addition to getting your body ready, getting your mind and spirit ready are just as essential for conception. Stress can create chemicals in the body that act like toxins and can fatigue the hormone system. Exercise, meditation and deep breathing are essential to reducing stress, and will help men and women be in a more balanced and receptive mood for conception.

When getting ready for pregnancy, imagine a sacred place you would like to see your child growing and developing. Do you imagine this space as supportive, nutritive, relaxing, and balanced? Realize that you can create this place for your child within yourself and your environment. Becoming pregnant in a depleted and imbalanced state can be a contributing factor to infertility and complications during pregnancy.

A healthy relationship with your partner, and with your own body, can be very empowering during this time period. Keeping a journal can help you reflect, look towards the future, and keep you motivated about your health. Make a commitment not only to yourself, but also to your partner and your unborn baby, to add wellness and balance into your life. You are worth it!

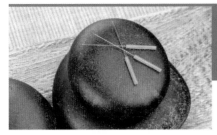

Acupuncture for Fertility

By Dr. Adrienne Stewart

Traditional Chinese Medicine (TCM) has been addressing infertility for thousands of years with safe and effective treatments. Practitioners use acupuncture for fertility to help balance the body's overall system. Acupuncture is the use of very thin, sterile needles placed strategically along the body to help balance the flow of energy that Chinese medicine calls Qi. Because TCM sees illness as an imbalance in the body's energy system, it focuses on treating the whole person rather than the symptoms. Using acupuncture for pregnancy is about restoring balance to the body's overall system, thus increasing fertility naturally. Women often turn to acupuncture for fertility because it is gentle and effective, does not put mother or baby at risk, and helps overall wellness.

Fertility and acupuncture have been linked topics in mainstream medicine since studies began revealing that conventional treatments such as in vitro fertilization (IVF) are enhanced when combined with acupuncture. In one study, women who underwent IVF treatment in combination with acupuncture before and after fertilized eggs were transferred to their uterus, were much more likely to get pregnant from the procedure. Research has also shown that using acupuncture for fertility can stimulate egg production in women who can't or don't want to use fertility medications. Acupuncture can also address some underlying causes of infertility as well as stimulate follicular function, hormone balancing, and blood flow.

To receive the best results when using acupuncture for pregnancy, it is important to maintain consistent treatment over an extended period of time. Treatment with acupuncture should start several months before conventional treatments. If using acupuncture alone for fertility, patients need to keep in mind that it may take time to stimulate the body to heal and come into balance. Because acupuncture is so safe, it can be used long into pregnancy to help prevent miscarriage. In addition, acupuncture can also be used to stimulate labor when a woman is overdue. Whether used alone or in combination with conventional treatments, acupuncture for fertility is sure to improve the chances for a successful pregnancy.

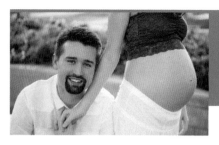

Confessions from the Pregnant Doctor

By Dr. Adrienne Stewart

I am currently in the last few weeks of pregnancy, and I have learned so much! Now that I have experienced pregnancy myself, I can tell you that it is completely different than what the textbooks said. There are times when my "doctor self" knows what to do, whereas other times my "first-time pregnant self" is asking, "WHAT IN THE WORLD IS GOING ON?!"

By sharing my experience, I hope to provide some comfort to those who are struggling with feeling their best. I also want to let pregnant women know they are not alone!

Pregnancy & the BODY
There are many changes in the body! It is true that hormonal ups and downs are no joke!

For the first half of pregnancy, I really struggled with nausea and fatigue. I would wake up dry heaving or throwing up. After getting ready for work and pushing through the work day, I would often dry heave again on my one-hour commute back home. In the evenings and on weekends, I was either on the couch, in the bathroom, or in bed. Running errands or doing anything else was nearly impossible. Experiencing this day after day and week after week got depressing. I would often wake up thinking how I just wanted the day to be over and to fall back asleep. This was a completely new feeling for me, because I'm used to being able to do the things I want to do. I now have a new appreciation for feeling healthy, and a deeper compassion for my patients that come in telling me they just want to feel like themselves again.

Therapies that have helped me address these physical issues included naturopathic care (of course), acupuncture, prenatal massage, craniosacral therapy, and pregnancy-focused chiropractic care. I have to admit that certain therapies would help at some times and not others. I am a huge proponent of taking good quality supplements, but there were times that, as soon as I put them in my mouth, they would just come back up. I felt guilty at times because my "doctor self" knows how important they are, and yet my "pregnant self" would just say, "Yeah, right." This solidifies for me why pre-conceptive and preventative care is so important. Building up the body by providing it with great nutrients and eliminating toxins provides the foundation for the body to flourish. Then, when we have life stressors, obstacles, or illness, our bodies can overcome them or have the resilience to get back on track more readily.

Pregnancy & the MIND
The first symptom I had of pregnancy was "pregnancy brain." I forgot my appointment for a massage and knew something must be off. It wasn't like me, and I sure needed that massage! Throughout pregnancy, I learned that I just needed to write things down and make sure I kept a calendar. There would be times when someone would tell me something and, 30 minutes later, I would forget what we were talking about. If this happens to you (whether you are pregnant or not), don't beat yourself up. When I could just let it be without judging myself or stressing about it, I would later remember.

The other mental and hormonal change that I should mention is crying very easily or for no particular reason. I have told my patients that if they start crying, I am likely to join them. There are also times that my husband comes home and finds me "ugly crying," and we both start laughing because I don't even know the reason. So, if this ever happens to you, try to not take yourself too seriously and have a good laugh about it.

Pregnancy & the SPIRIT
Even though I am very much ready for my baby to be in my arms and for this pregnancy to be at the end, I have to say that this experience has been the best time of my life. I've never felt so special. In times of vulnerability, I asked for help and let go of my perceived control. Plus, I have a new purpose and responsibility in life. In the end, the power of a woman's body, my bond with my husband, and the strong love I feel for my baby whom I haven't even met yet, have all deepened my awareness of how beautiful life truly is!

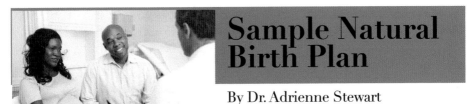

Sample Natural Birth Plan
By Dr. Adrienne Stewart

Several patients and friends have asked me what a birth plan is, and what an example looks like. Basically, a birth plan is how you envision your labor and delivery. It's important to realize that you have options, whether you are having a hospital birth or an at-home birth. By writing down a plan ahead of time, you don't have to worry about some of these decisions when it is time for birth. I am including a natural birth plan that is very similar to the one I used for my daughter's birth. Feel free to modify with your preferences.

Mother's Name
Date of Birth
Name of OB or Midwife
We would like the following people to be present for the birth of our baby:
_____. We understand that complications do arise and in such instances trust
our midwife/doctor to communicate what is involved in making the necessary
decisions. We greatly appreciate your cooperation in realizing our plan.

Environment
I would like the nurses and staff to please talk softly, compassionately, and
explain every procedure, no matter how routine.

Considering we will have several people in the room, please limit the amount
of extra personnel in the room.

Prep
Vaginal Exams: I prefer minimal vaginal examinations if my water has broken.

Amniotic Sac: I prefer to allow the amniotic sac to break naturally.

Group B Strep: If positive for GBS, IV antibiotics are preferred.

Labor
Interventions: As long as our baby and I are healthy, we would prefer no
interventions that are not medically necessary.

Medications: We would like to try to avoid all medications during birth.

Please don't offer; we will ask if wanted. I would prefer no IVs unless
medically necessary. If needed, I prefer a heparin lock.

Food and Water: I want the option to eat and drink during labor if desired.

Inducing: If our labor slows or stalls and my baby and I are both well, we will
decline a chemical induction and prefer using homeopathy or acupressure.

Positions for Labor: I would like the freedom to change positions, stand or
walk around, use the birth ball, or sit in the labor tub as desired.

Episiotomy: I prefer to have no episiotomy and risk tearing. To prevent
tearing, please apply almond/olive oil or warm water compresses to soften
the perineum.

Delivery
I would like to view the birth using a mirror.

_____ would like the option to catch our baby if possible.

I would like our baby to be placed immediately skin-to-skin on my chest.

Cord Clamping: I would like to delay cord clamping until the cord stops
pulsating completely. _____ will cut the cord.

I would prefer not to have Pitocin after delivery unless I am losing too much blood.

Newborn Procedures

Please inform us of all procedures, no matter how routine.

We would like to postpone any routine newborn procedures until we have had a chance to bond with our baby and after our baby has successfully breastfed.

Cleaning: We do not want our baby to be wiped down immediately after birth. Please keep vernix on the skin.

Breastfeeding: Breastfeeding is very important to us. We would like to decline any artificial nipples, pacifiers, formula or supplements for our baby.

Hepatitis B vaccine and antibiotic eye drops: We would like to approve/decline the Hep B vaccine and approve/decline prophylactic eye antibiotics. We plan to discuss these with our pediatrician. We would like to sign the waiver ahead of time.

Vitamin K: We would prefer the vitamin K injection be given after breastfeeding and bonding, unless medically necessary.

PKU: Please do routine PKU testing after 24 hours.

Circumcision: We do/do not want our baby boy to be circumcised.

We would like to take home the placenta.

We prefer that our hospital stay be as short as possible.

In Case of Emergency

If the situation warrants, we would prefer a vacuum extraction to a cesarean.

Cesarean: We would like to avoid a cesarean if at all possible, unless it is necessary for the wellbeing of mother or baby and all other options have been exhausted.

I would like my husband to be present at all times during the operation.

I would like to be conscious and informed of all pre- and postoperative medications. I prefer no sedatives after birth and non-drowsy anti-nausea medications if possible.

I would like the urine catheter to be inserted after my anesthesia so I do not feel it.

I would like the screen lowered once my baby's head is out so that I can see the birth.

I would like to have immediate contact with our baby and breastfeed as soon as possible. While suturing my skin back, I would like our baby to be placed on my chest or _____'s chest.

I prefer a double layer uterine closure to allow for a successful VBAC with future pregnancies.

If our baby has any problems, I would like _____ to be present at all times.

Thank You!

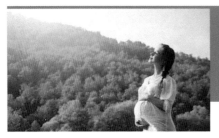

Affirmations During Pregnancy & Labor

By Dr. Adrienne Stewart

Affirmations can help people stay optimistic and feel empowered, especially through transitions in life. You can create your own personal affirmations or use the sample affirmations that resonate best with you. Pregnancy and staying strong in labor can be very challenging.

I recommend writing affirmations down and hanging them throughout your house on mirrors or on the refrigerator where you will see them regularly. You may also want to bring a few to hang in the delivery room. Personally, I used some of the following affirmations to help me stay positive and strong in the last few weeks of my pregnancy and during labor.

My baby is happy and healthy

My body knows how to have this baby, just as my body knew how to grow this baby

I am ready and prepared for childbirth

I can handle the pain

I am STRONG

Each contraction brings my baby closer

I am patient and relaxed

My baby will arrive at the perfect time

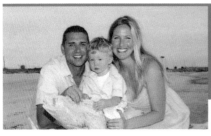

Keeping Fit and Healthy with Your Kids!

By Dr. Linda Khoshaba

Preventative health in children is an important topic to focus on, as this can set the foundation for optimal lifelong health. Teaching kids to eat right and stay active can implement lasting values and help prevent disease. Here are some simple tips to help keep you and your family fit, healthy, and having fun!

Healthy Eating

Since kids spend a majority of their time at school, making sure that they are getting their essential nutrients from a diet dense in antioxidants, protein and good sources of carbohydrates and fats is extremely important. Packing a lunch that contains these key ingredients can have tremendous impact in the long term. This will also help curb cravings, especially for those high calorie foods that look delicious behind the vending machine glass. When it comes to snacks, great ideas include organic celery stalks with nut butters, fruit kabobs, hummus and veggies. Avoid the sugary drinks! Instead, try some water with lemon to make light lemonade!

Healthy Living

We live in a society that is bombarded with electronics, ranging from computers, tablets and hand held devices to other media sources. Naturally, our children have become experts at using them. The average screen time for children is approximately 3 hours per day. The downside is that there is a direct correlation between the amount of screen time and obesity. Therefore, limiting the duration and using this time for high quality content would be extremely beneficial in reducing factors that contribute to obesity, including a high BMI (Body Mass Index). Try balancing screen time with some lean time. Lean time is related to physical activity such as playing sports, walking outdoors, dancing and swimming.

> # Healthy Living
>
> The average screen time for children is approximately 3 hours per day. The downside is that there is a direct correlation between the amount of screen time and obesity.

Healthy Body

The best medicine is preventative medicine. Childhood years are extremely important in educating and bringing awareness to the negative consequences associated with tobacco and recreational drug and alcohol use. Being a positive role model is significant. Focus on creating a healthy body image by complimenting children on their efforts and accomplishments. This positive feedback will increase their overall self esteem. It is important to discuss healthy body messages and overcome the media pressure created by "ideal" images for both girls and boys.

Healthy Mind and Spirit

Helping and guiding children through mental and emotional health behaviors is as important as addressing physical needs.

Healthy Mind and Spirit
Helping and guiding children through mental and emotional health behaviors is as important as addressing physical needs. Whether it is related to temper tantrums or going through puberty, having a supportive family and friends can help improve the development process. Some great ways to improve this area include finding time for spiritual practices, meditation and relaxation. This is a wonderful way to get kids involved in the community and challenges them to learn a new hobby or skill.

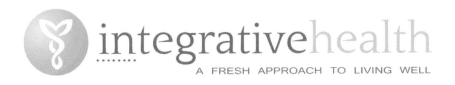

integrative health

A FRESH APPROACH TO LIVING WELL

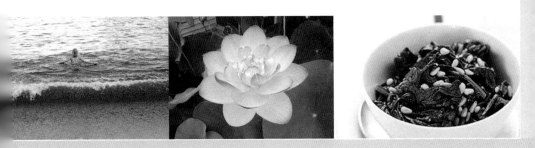

Resources

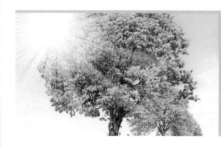

Want More from Integrative Health?

Office Visits:
Call our office at 480-657-0003.
Visit our website at
www.myintegrativehealth.com

Newsletter:
Sign up on our homepage:
www.myintegrativehealth.com

Podcast:
Getting Fresh With Your Health
Available in iTunes

App:
HypoThyroid App:
www.hypothyroidapp.com
Available in App Store

YouTube Channel:
Integrative Health: A Fresh
Approach to Living Well

Facebook:
Integrative Health: In Good Health

Twitter:
Integrative Health: In Good Health

Pinterest:
www.pinterest.com/
IHInGoodHealth

Books:
Healing Hashimoto's
*The Complete Idiot's Guide to
Thyroid Disease*

Online Programs:
www.ihmarketplace.com

Made in the USA
Charleston, SC
02 July 2014